The Invisible Smile
Living without facial expression

The Invisible Smile
Living without facial expression

Jonathan Cole
with Henrietta Spalding

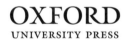
OXFORD
UNIVERSITY PRESS

OXFORD
UNIVERSITY PRESS

Great Clarendon Street, Oxford OX2 6DP

Oxford University Press is a department of the University of Oxford.
It furthers the University's objective of excellence in research, scholarship,
and education by publishing worldwide in

Oxford New York

Auckland Cape Town Dar es Salaam Hong Kong Karachi
Kuala Lumpur Madrid Melbourne Mexico City Nairobi
New Delhi Shanghai Taipei Toronto

With offices in

Argentina Austria Brazil Chile Czech Republic France Greece
Guatemala Hungary Italy Japan Poland Portugal Singapore
South Korea Switzerland Thailand Turkey Ukraine Vietnam

Oxford is a registered trade mark of Oxford University Press
in the UK and in certain other countries

Published in the United States
by Oxford University Press Inc., New York

© Oxford University Press 2009

A catalogue record for this title is available from the British Library
Data available

Library of Congress Cataloguing in Publication Data
Data available

Typeset by Cepha Imaging Private Ltd., Bangalore, India
Printed in Great Britain
on acid-free paper by
Biddles Ltd., King's Lynn, Norfolk

ISBN 978–0–19–856639–7

10 9 8 7 6 5 4 3 2 1

The word is to the thought as the feeling is to the facial expression.

Charles Bell

Imagining what it is like to be someone other than yourself is at the core of our humanity. It is the essence of compassion, and the beginning of morality.

Ian McEwan, *The Observer*, July 2005

To those who allowed us a glimpse inside their Möbius
and
for those who live with a visible, or invisible difference.

Acknowledgements

Jonathan Cole

This work was driven by curiosity and indignation. I had first met Möbius syndrome when writing what I called a 'natural history of the face', which I approached by going to ask those who have a problem with use of the face about their experience; hence my calling it also 'an unnatural history'. I wrote about a man who, blinded as an adult, had been depressed not when his sight faded but when his precious visual memories of his loved ones faded, since then, at that time, he had no other way to represent them. I wrote about those with acquired disfigurement and the stigma they faced. Within this there were two short narratives of those with Möbius syndrome who live without being able to show facial expression. But though these stories fitted with my overall work, I was well aware that I had not encompassed the experience of Möbius Syndrome with any depth.

Henrietta, who lives with Möbius, had read my book and was indignant that I had featured her condition so starkly and cursorily. She phoned me up out of the blue and attacked (in the gentlest and most constructive way imaginable). I was delighted, and rather than defend my work suggested we collaborate on a fuller account of this condition. To her credit, she agreed.

Our aim was to divide the work evenly, in the hope that my relative experience of writing might complement her first hand knowledge of Möbius. We agreed immediately that since medical aspects of the condition were already known, what was needed was an account of the subjective experience of living without facial movement.

Soon after this Henrietta became ill, with a problem unrelated to Möbius. This meant that though she had conducted three interviews, her ability to do more was reduced. So I have done the other interviews together with the writing and editing. Fortunately, Henrietta bounced back and has been involved at all stages, directing me towards the people to interview, reading and rereading drafts, and guiding me as my ideas developed. Our aim was to produce a work by two people where the authorship of each part was seamless. We hope to have achieved that in a different way, but one which has been dependent on Henrietta throughout. My first and greatest acknowledgement is, therefore, to her. To go with me on a journey deep into her own condition was not always easy. Her humour and resourcefulness were a continuing inspiration.

Our thanks are due next to all who agreed to take part in open-ended interviews, often over days. All did so with candour and sensitivity; I hope we have repaid their trust. All have also approved their accounts.

We must also thank Linda Anderson and the UK Moebius Syndrome Support Group and especially Vicki McCarrell and the US Moebius Syndrome Foundation for their assistance and support. In particular, the Foundation supported my recent visit to Bethesda, and Vicki has been as brilliant and encouraging to us as she is to all the people with Möbius in the USA and throughout the world. Changing Faces in London has given us the use of its offices at various times as well as acting as a spiritual home and we thank James Partridge, its director, for this and much more.

I am grateful to Rhonda Robert, Bencie Woll, and Roger Baker for their advice in scientific matters outside my usual areas and to Sue Sutherland, Chief Executive of Poole Hospital Foundation NHS Trust, for employing me in my day job and for offering implicit support for my eccentricity of writing. Alfredo Fernández was kind enough to allow us to reproduce his drawings. I am also very grateful to The MIT Press for allowing me to reproduce parts of my book *About Face* in this work: in particular, the chapter 'The spectator' (p. 67–73) is a reduced version of a chapter in that book.

We are grateful to Oxford University Press for publishing this work and, in particular, to Martin Baum for his support and encouragement, especially during its early commissioning stage. From that time our thanks are also due to Shaun Gallagher and Dan Zahavi for supporting personal, first-person experiences within neuroscience.

At OUP, Carol Maxwell, Alison Lees, Joanna Hardern, and Marionne Cronin were all enormously helpful in various aspects of the book's production; their care, attention to detail, and lightness of touch were much appreciated.

I must also, as ever, thank my wife Sue for her enduring and un-wavering support in a myriad of ways. To be married to a full-time doctor, at a time when he is old enough to have more administrative and political duties come his way, must be bad enough, but to have one who insists on writing as well must be an order of magnitude worse.

For her part, Henrietta would like to thank her mother and father for their support and love.

Lastly she wants to acknowledge that, for her and all with Möbius, there is no such word as can't.

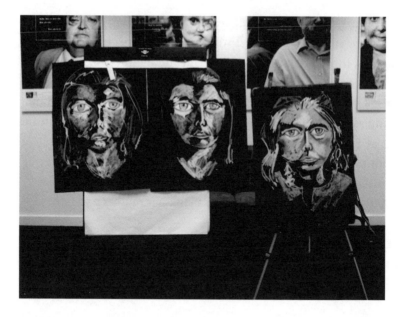

Three portraits of Henrietta Spalding, by Alfredo Fernandez

Left: One morning in Berlin
Middle: The afternoon in Berlin
Right: Some months later in London

See Chapter 9 for details

Contents

Chapter 1

Introduction

The 5-year-old boy looked up at his father and asked,

'Why can't I be happy?'

His father had no reply. His son, Josh, had Möbius[1] syndrome, a condition in which children are born without movement of the face and facial expression. Josh was clearly relating facial movement to the inner experience of emotion. He thought people were happy because they smiled, and since he could not smile, he reasoned, he could not be happy.[2]

We human beings have defined ourselves at various times by our upright posture, opposable thumb and finger, tool use, speech and language, cognitive power, and even by our aggression. But we are also unique in having a mobile expressive face, which gives a read-out of our feelings and emotions[3] as we communicate and converse. We are, perhaps above all, highly social and yet highly individual; our faces are both individual identifiers and communicators of our inner states. This was brought home to me, some years ago, when I saw an elderly lady who had lost facial expression as a result of a rare stroke syndrome. At a clinical meeting many thought her demented, not because she behaved oddly but because she could not respond to questions with changes in her facial expression. Just as deaf meant 'dumb', unable to speak and so unable to think, so facial inanimation and impassivity was interpreted as meaning cognitive absence.

We look entranced at a newborn baby; mother and child spend hours of 'face time' together. Later we lose ourselves in our lovers' faces. In politics we face down the opposition, hoping to blink second. John Hull, who went blind as an adult, became most depressed not when he lost sight but when the visual memories of his loved ones' faces faded [Cole, 1998]. Faces, to an extent, define us.

In one of his last essays Merleau-Ponty [1964*a*] wrote that, 'Science manipulates things and gives up living in them.' Empirical science; measurement, experimentation, confirmation and falsification of hypothesis, asking nature questions, is perhaps the most powerful tool for understanding the world around us, and is also supremely stimulating, enjoyable, and enthralling. But such a view, from the outside of 'things', can find it difficult to capture the subjective experience of chronic neurological impairment; what it is like to live with something, day in, day out, and from birth. Then, what is needed is the witness of those who, in Merleau-Ponty's phrase, 'live in' the impairment.

The heart of this book is a series of narratives which explore what it is like to live with Möbius and, therefore, without facial movement and facial expression. Also, living with the other less obvious problems associated with the condition, and the effects this has on one as a child or an adult. A dozen or more people with Möbius syndrome discuss their childhood, adolescence, and adult lives, their schooling and jobs, personal relationships, and reactions to meeting new people. Though the perspective of these narratives is from the inside of Möbius, it does allow reflections on what most of us take from granted; what the face does and how it defines us. Though Möbius syndrome is very rare, with around 0.002% of births from a sample in The Netherlands,[4] and just one of many abnormalities of cranial nerve and craniofacial development, it is our contention that by looking at the consequences of living without facial movement we can learn something of what the face does in us all in a manner, and to a depth, not possible in other ways.

Though the most obvious feature of Möbius syndrome is the absence of movement of the muscles of facial expression, the condition actually has many more and differing features. These will now be considered in clinical terms; if you prefer not to know too much about this aspect then please rejoin at 'Inside Möbius' (p. 8).

Möbius unmasked

The cardinal features of Möbius are two; congenital palsies of the VIth and VIIth cranial nerves. The VIth, the abducens, is necessary for outward movement, or abduction, of the eyes. People with Möbius, therefore, cannot move the eyes outwards or from side to side horizontally.

Since many movements of the eyes involve some abduction, from tracking something moving to fixating on an object further away when the eyes diverge, people with Möbius have problems with vision in many differing ways and learn to turn their heads to look at something rather than try to move their eyes in their sockets. The VIIth cranial nerve, the facial, controls the movements of the muscles of facial expression. These include those around the eyes, and mouth, nose, and forehead. There are a few muscles supplied by another cranial nerve, the Vth, or trigeminal, which are involved with jaw movement and eating, notably the temporalis and masseter, which are not affected, but these are not involved in expression. The absence of movement of the facial muscles means that those muscles tend to atrophy, giving the face a characteristic rather smooth look, with open mouth. But there is a range of visible differences. I once asked at a conference what a man with Möbius that I wanted to meet, looked like. Someone said that he looked like me. And he did, gaunt with thinning, greying hair. Some have more obvious Möbius, possibly because of associated cranial conditions.

The first person to describe this combination of palsies was von Graefe [1880]. After this there were several further descriptions of the condition before Paul Julius Möbius reviewed three subjects with congenital non-progressive bilateral facial and abducens palsy; since then the syndrome has borne his name.[5]

In the intervening years there have been a number of studies refining the syndrome, with differing criteria for inclusion, but the two main problems, facial weakness or paralysis and eye abduction, are essential for the diagnosis. In one recent paper from the Dutch group [Verzijl et al., 2003] 37 subjects were assessed. Of these 97% had bilateral facial weakness and the remaining 3% a unilateral weakness. This weakness was complete in 34% whilst in the majority, 62%, there was relative sparing of the lower part of the face, including the muscles around the mouth and the platysma muscle; a thin sheet which sits beneath the jaw over the anterior neck. Though paralysis of abduction of the eyes is a cardinal feature, the abnormalities of eye movement were frequently more complex than this. Crossed eyes, or esotropia, were seen in 19 subjects bilaterally and one crossed eye in four subjects. In contrast, in 9% the eyes pointed abnormally outwards. All subjects were unable to abduct the eyes beyond the midline, while a further 17 subjects had difficulties in moving the eyes together; a horizontal gaze paresis. Duane syndrome, a complex disorder comprising limited abduction, and adduction of the eyes with retraction (deepening) of the eye with narrowing of the eyelid by the nose, was seen in 34%. Fibrosis of the muscles that move the eye was seen in 9%, further restricting their movement.

Verzijl et al. found that 77% of their sample also had a small tongue, which in some was asymmetrical. Feeding problems at birth were seen in 32 subjects, due to insufficient sucking, defects of swallowing, and weakness of the palatal muscles or regurgitation. A further six had some weakness of biting due to a Vth cranial nerve problem and 29% had some degree of hearing loss. Most also had abnormalities of craniofacial development, with 89% having folds at the nasal side of the eye (epicanthic folds), 81% a flattened nasal bridge, 64% a small jaw, 61% a high arched palate, 47% external ear abnormalities, and 33% teeth problems.

Möbius is not only a face thing. In this sample, seven had difficulties in breathing at birth and two died of this. Of the remaining five, there were persistent breathing and heart rhythm difficulties for years. Thirty-one subjects also had some malformation of their arms or legs, with missing fingers, reduced muscle development of the calves and extremely high arched feet (talipes). Absence or underdevelopment of the breast muscle, pectoralis, was seen in four subjects (Poland syndrome).

Of the sample of 34 subjects tested all but four also had problems with movement. Twenty-three showed late development of standing and sitting, difficulties in running, jumping, and hopping, and poor finer skills. None could dance, do gymnastics, or play a musical instrument. A majority, 82%, were clumsy and three used a tricycle rather than a bicycle because of this. Lastly there is evidence in the literature of learning difficulties and autism associated with Möbius, though the incidence of these varies quite markedly between groups. Thus, learning problems, or mental retardation as it is described in some papers, has rates of 33–75% by some [Cronemberger et al., 2001; Gillberg and

Steffenburg, 1989; Johansson *et al.*, 2001] but only 5% by another. [Verzijl *et al.*, 2005*a*] Autism has similar wide ranges of incidence from published samples, from 5–40%. [Bandim *et al.*, 2003; Cronemberger *et al.*, 2001; Gillberg and Steffenburg, 1989; Miller *et al.*, 2005; Strömland *et al.*, 2002; Verzijl *et al.*, 2005*a*] Though the consensus is that Möbius syndrome is associated with various cognitive problems, the precise frequency of these is unclear.

The fact that the above abnormalities of cranial nerves, coordination, and limb development are seen to differing degrees in different people suggests that rather than Möbius being a precise, predetermined syndrome it might better be called a sequence, implying varying symptoms and varying degrees of expression in the bodily phenotype. Though there is general agreement about this within medical workers, since this work is not directed primarily towards clinicians and scientists, we will use the more widely known and accepted term syndrome.

The where and why of Möbius

The simplest way of explaining all these various abnormalities is to suggest that the problem lies in an area of the brain, called the lower brainstem, which lies underneath the main structures of the brain just above the spinal cord. This region develops from a single embryological origin, and it is, therefore, considered that Möbius is primarily a developmental disorder of this area, called the rhomboencephalon, though with limb maldevelopment as well, it is clear that the problem is widespread. It is presumed that the clumsiness and movement problems are due to involvement of the long tracts of nerve cells through which the brain controls movement, which travel through the brain stem so, within this area, this is not simply a cranial-nerve problem. This is important since it distances Möbius from a collection of cranial-nerve problems collectively known as the congenital cranial dysinnervation disorders (CCDDs) and more specifically from a similar condition, hereditary congenital facial palsy, which affects the VIIth nerve alone.

Evidence for Möbius being a brain-stem problem comes from a variety of workers including reviews of post-mortem, neurophysiological, and imaging studies by Verzijl *et al.* [2005*b*; 2005*c*; 2005*d*]. They conclude that there may be four differing types of pathology: maldevelopment of the nerves of the cranial nerve nuclei in the lower brainstem; degeneration of nerves more distally in the facial and other nerves; more widespread scarring of wide areas of the brainstem; and, lastly, a peripheral form in which the problem may be in the muscle rather than in the nerves or nerve nuclei.[6]

The cause, or causes, of Möbius have been considered since its first description and remain unresolved. There are three main theories: that it is a consequence of a genetic, chromosomal problem; that it is due to a problem in vascular supply to the baby during pregnancy in the womb; and that it is a consequence of an environmental toxin.

Most cases of Möbius are sporadic and do not run in families, suggesting that if this is a genetic condition then the penetrance is very low or that the condition is caused by a spontaneous mutation. There is a very low risk for siblings and several cases have been described in one of a set of (non-identical) twins. In those cases in which there is a clearer family history no single gene defect has been found responsible. In various studies abnormalities of chromosomes 13 (13q12.2-13) [Ziter *et al.*, 1991], 1 (1p22) [Donahue *et al.*, 1993], 3 (3q21-22) [Kremer *et al.*, 1996], and 10 (10q21.3-22.1) [Verzijl *et al.*, 1999] have been described. Other conditions with overlapping problems, such as the CCDDs and Duane's, have other chromosomal abnormalities. It seems that we are some way from understanding any genetic cause for Möbius, likely though this seems. There may be differing subtypes of Möbius and, in common with other conditions, a single chromosomal abnormality may be unlikely.

The next stage is to probe what the genes on a particular chromosome might do. In looking at Möbius, which is a movement or motor problem primarily, rather than a sensory one, one must consider how these neurones might develop. Elisabeth Engle, at a recent meeting on Möbius,[7] suggested that movement or motor neurones have to develop in the embryo, find the right location, involving a significant migratory pathway, and then send out dendrites to connect to other cells. One of these dendrites has to become polarized to form its main trunk or axon and this then has to find its appropriate target and develop the right branches. These steps are poorly understood in neurobiology in general though some progress is being made in various rare CCDDs and other conditions that may be relevant to Möbius.

'HOX' genes are conserved across many animal species and are involved in segmentation and development. In a small population of consanguineous people, in several parts of the world, defects in expression of HOX genes have been found to result in limb deformities and in horizontal gaze abnormalities, deafness, facial weakness, hypoventilation, vascular malformations of the internal carotid arteries and cardiac outflow tract, mental retardation, and autism spectrum disorder. [Tischfield *et al.*, 2005] Such a HOX gene defect has not yet been found in people with Möbius, but may be of relevance.

Similarly another gene, ROBO3, which is known to be important for nerve axon guidance in a variety of species, including *Drosophila* fruit fly and zebra fish, appears to be involved in allowing motor axons to develop during intrauterine development in man [Jen *et al.*, 2004]. In the rare condition of horizontal gaze palsy with progressive scoliosis, both motor and sensory nerves seem uncrossed. Since much of this crossing takes place in the brainstem, the area affected in Möbius, this finding may be useful in Möbius. As yet, however, this work is a beginning and nothing more.

A second theory about the causes of Möbius is that it reflects a deleterious vascular event in the womb, which affects the baby's blood supply to the brain during early pregnancy. Bavinck and Weaver [1986] suggested that between the fourth and sixth week of gestation one artery supplying the brain stem, the subclavian, might be particularly vulnerable to obstruction or delayed development, whether due to a mechanical, genetic, or environmental cause. An alternative theory is that perfusion of the brain in this area fails because of what is called watershed insufficiency between the circulation areas of two separate arteries [Sarnat, 2004]. Though the Dutch group are critical of this theory, not least since it does not explain the frequent limb malformations, others are more enthusiastic and offer support from studies of people born with Möbius after increased bleeding during early pregnancy and use of drugs that are known to cause constriction of the blood vessels of the uterus (see below).

This theory does not exclude a genetic cause since it is possible than there is a genetic susceptibility to arterial insufficiency, though this has not been proved as yet. It is also the case that exposure to certain drugs by the mother in the early weeks of pregnancy, which can lead to subsequent Möbius in the baby, might act through vascular insufficiency. This has been reported after exposure to cocaine [Hoyne *et al.*, 1990] and ergotamine [Hughes and Goldstein, 1988], for instance. The main evidence for this theory, however, comes from Brazil where the drug misoprostol, a synthetic prostaglandin E1 analogue, is used to induce abortion [Gonzalez *et al.*, 1993; Pastuszak, *et al.*, 1998; Vargas *et al.*, 2000], when used with methotrexate and mifepristone.[8] Pastuszak *et al.* [1998] compared mothers of babies with Möbius with mothers of children with a neural-tube defect, as a way of establishing whether misoprostol was specifically associated with the former condition. Among the mothers of 96 infants with Möbius' syndrome, 47 (49%) had used misoprostol in the first trimester of pregnancy, as compared with 3 (3%) of the mothers of 96 infants with neural-tube defects.

Möbius syndrome, then, may not have a single cause, and even identifiable causes may interrelate; for example, in post-mortem examinations of three children exposed to misoprostol, vascular damage to the brain was shown [Marques-Dias *et al.*, 2003]. In most sporadic cases, however, no clear drug or vascular cause has been found, and it seems likely that a genetic problem may underpin them.

Inside Möbius

Necessary though it is to have clinical details, and Harriëtte Verzijl's doctoral thesis [2005] is probably the best collection of such data, neither a scientific approach, whether genetic or neurophysiological, nor clinical work, with its necessary focus on correcting deficits and impairments, is sufficient to understand what it is like to live with – and inside – Möbius. A human, first-person, subjective experience of Möbius is important to allow us to understand the condition and so help those with it more. But, important though this is, it might have limited appeal. What the stories of those with Möbius reveal is something of how the face helps define our sense of self and our social being. It is within the narratives of these people that we learn about what we take for granted – a mobile expressive face – and the remainder of the book is, therefore, concerned with such narratives.

In the first chapter, 'Someone home' (p. 13–23), the first few days and months of living with Möbius are related. This is, necessarily, from the parents' perspective and is largely concerned with the practicalities of looking after a small baby with such a condition. But it is also about their thoughts and feelings when faced with such an unexpected event.

Once the first frantic days are over, with a myriad of medical opinion and appointments, then come the early childhood years and school. Children with Möbius have a range of problems to cope with and require immense and continuing support from parents, teachers, and many other workers. Gemma's story is given as an illustration of how this can work to give a child as normal a childhood as possible and, equally importantly, to allow her to develop to her maximal capacity. This, too, is largely told from the perspective of her parents.

In the next chapter, in contrast, an adult with Möbius looks back to her childhood and how she viewed herself as a child. Her body constantly let her down, whether because of her eyesight, feeding problems, or walking. In contrast, even as a young child, she knew she was bright. So stark was this difference between body and mind that she felt her self, her being, her Celia, to be within her mind and not in her body. This led not only to altered relations with others but also a curious reduction in the way she felt emotion. In this chapter, others, including a young boy called Duncan, with similar and overlapping experiences of childhood, are also met, as this relation between facial movement and expression, and emotional communication is first explored.

We then progress to consider the reflections and narratives of four adults with Möbius. Lizzie is a young adult and the only person featured to have a one-sided facial palsy. She also has an unaffected twin sister. Lizzie reflects on her school progress and just how much effort she has had to put in to succeed. She had to repeat years several times and each time was left behind by her hard-won friends. She also discusses her meetings with others with Möbius and the advantages and disadvantages of this.

In 'The spectator' (p. 67–73), we meet someone in his fifties who only found out his diagnosis about ten years ago. James was late going to school and yet ten years later had won a place at Cambridge. Despite these considerable achievements he relates a somewhat similar experience to Celia in that he has spent much of his time in a life of the mind:

> 'I think I get trapped in my mind or my head. I sort of *think* happy or I *think* sad, not really saying or recognizing actually feeling happy or feeling sad. Perhaps I have had a difficulty in recognizing that which I'm putting a name to is not a thought at all but it is a feeling; maybe I have to intellectualize mood.'

In the next chapter Alison and her mother tell two sides of the same story. She is in her late forties and has learning problems and Möbius associated with eyelids that droop over her eyes; a condition called ptosis. The effects of these on her life and on those of her family become clear.

Last in this section, Matthew tells his story. He is the only person to be using his own name, but then he is sufficiently well known from several TV appearances and from his work within the Möbius community in the USA that anonymity would be difficult to maintain. He has, over years, offered his experiences to younger people with Möbius and worked with scientists on aspects of face and emotion recognition. Here the possibilities of a longer personal narrative allow him to express his experiences and situation in more depth than he may have done previously.

In Chapter 9 we leave accounts of Möbius for a short visit to Berlin, and for Henrietta's and my own single appearance. I had been asked to lecture there and was then asked if I would bring a patient along too, whose portrait would be drawn in front of a group of medical students. Our aim, in agreeing, was to make people more aware of facial visible difference, and to undermine a purely visual way of looking at people. Our reasoning was that with Möbius one had to look beyond the face since it showed so little. As will be seen, things did not work out quite as we expected.

In the last three narrative chapters we return to the experience of Möbius. Each of these people has had a remarkable journey, not only with the condition but in gaining insights into the experience of emotion, which some with Möbius find so problematic. Eleanor remembers her time as a teenager and then at university. Like Celia, she hardly knew emotion as a child and had a pretty miserable adolescence. But once at university she was amongst people who cared less about appearance and more about her. It gave her a chance to mould her character anew and so she set about watching others and taking from each what she liked:

> 'I wanted to be someone who people would like. Before, people had not liked me, so I wanted to be sweet, gentle, and likeable. I did not want to be radical – at the time there were lots like that. I did not want to stand out. I just wanted to be inoffensive, reliable, and so that is what I became.'

In 'Every second of the day' (p. 133–149), Cate describes her life, thus far, through bullying and cruelty at school (from many, including her brother), to her discovery that she could sing, her time at the Royal Academy of Music, her singing career, and, latterly, her time as a wife and mother. It was through singing that she first connected with emotional experience and it is when singing that she feels strongest and most alive.

Like Eleanor, Lydia used the freedom at university to develop her character, but though she was successful there, she felt that she had learnt to imitate those around her to fit in. It was when she became a teacher in Spain, immersed in their richly expressive culture and embodied gesture, that she found she was not merely aping others but beginning to experience as well. In her own words, 'Because of the cultural up-regulation of feeling in gesture I learnt to feel ... I could feel really ecstatic, happy, for the first time ever.' Though she is unclear how she managed to bootstrap emotional experience within herself from bodily expressions, she is clear that it took the expansive gestures and social life of Spain. She returned the favour by assisting in the formation of a Spanish Möbius group and was soon helping them on the world stage.

The chapter 'Rusty old car' (p. 159–176) is reflective from the perspective of those with Möbius. We hear what it is like for one person living with Möbius and its limitations on a day-to-day basis. People with the condition discuss how concerns about intimacy and employment become more significant in the adult years and how resilience can be maintained.

Then, in the final chapter, more general themes are explored, beginning by returning to that puzzling difference in the literature in the incidence of learning difficulties and autism with Möbius. We then discuss the various problems that children with the condition may have in communication. A case is built up for communication between people being reliant not only on language and prosody of voice, or gesture and facial expression, but that all these, together, give differing information, which is combined to form the richness inherent in conversations with others. Those with Möbius show again and again the importance of the face in developing these and the consequences of loss. Then, finally we return to Duncan, who was first met as a boy and who is now a young man with a new son. This turns out to be a new beginning for both of them.

The challenges of Möbius vary between people and each person's response to these differs according to individuality and personality. But some of the challenges are shared. Sucking as a baby is often impossible, while eating and drinking remain difficult, since both need lips that close. Judging speeds, depth, and distances is often also difficult, with severe gaze palsies, meaning that the eyes may not move in their sockets and binocular vision develops poorly. For some, the facial difficulties are less onerous than those of the feet, with walking difficult and with chronic pain. People with Möbius also have to deal, often on a daily basis, with new people who stare and wonder. Though through speech therapy the diction of most people with Möbius has a miraculous clarity, to speak without being able to move the lips must be tiring. That your syndrome is named after a man whose name has two of the most difficult sounds for you to make – 'm' and 'b' – is just one of the ironies and unfair facts of life you have to rise above.

Chapter 2

Someone home

Parents usually recognize that something is wrong from birth, though it may be weeks, even years, before the word Möbius is met. Charlie outdid this; he was difficult before he was born, even before he was conceived.

Talipes

David and Lucy had decided that they wanted a second child, a sibling for 3-year-old Hugh, but they had problems conceiving. After months of trying they became despondent, starting to imagine their one-child family. They were about to start IVF when, after a trip abroad working, Lucy fell pregnant; they were so relieved.

At 14 weeks she bled, though a scan the next day showed that the baby was moving normally. A repeat scan at 20 weeks showed an abnormality of one foot, 'talipes'; they had no idea what it was; a kindly midwife provided lots of support and encouragement. But when she got home Lucy googled talipes on the web; 'One or both feet are twisted out of shape or into the wrong position. One of the main types, talipes equinovarus, is also known as club foot.' The search was terrifying, giving a long list of associated conditions, including learning difficulties. A scientist relative reassured them that talipes was quite common and that even athletes had been born with it. They still only told a few people; they did not want their unborn baby defined by a disability. Their obstetrician suggested an amniocentesis but they refused. As Catholics, terminating the pregnancy would have been difficult. In any case, Lucy wanted to enjoy her new baby as he grew; she did not want to focus on the negative. 'This child was just so wanted; talipes just didn't seem that bad ... '

Her labour began straightforwardly but then stalled and Lucy needed a Caesarean section. When the doctors gave Charlie to her, Lucy noticed something a little strange about his mouth. But then he was whisked off for assessment. Then, soon after, lots of people were looking at him. A junior doctor came up to say that Charlie had 'a syndrome', adding that there was something funny about his ears, and that he might have a hole in the heart. David fainted. Lucy immediately raced ahead to think about Charlie's care, his future and how they would manage.

David went home, mentioning to the family that there might be a few problems but did not dwell on it. The following day Lucy's mother visited. She just picked Charlie up and cuddled him, her normal reactions a welcome relief from all the clinical work around her.

Over the next few days a curious stream of doctors and students came to see Charlie, looking and prodding. Sometimes Lucy was told who they were, other times not. 'It looks like this …, it could be that,' the doctors were evidently busy leafing through a book of syndromes. Only one doctor stopped to ask how Lucy and David felt. Fortunately, no hole in the heart was found. Whilst the detective work went on they struggled to look after Charlie. He could not feed because his lips could not make a seal. The nurses encouraged them to use a bottle. But Lucy wanted him to have her milk so David brought in a breast pump and she expressed. It was time consuming but worth it.[1]

When finally they were allowed home, the next day they had to return to see the ophthalmologist. Tired and frightened, and with little idea of what all the appointments and consultants were for, they sat in a cold, draughty corridor surrounded by endless queues of other, anxious parents. They just wanted to be home getting to know Charlie. Afterwards they went home to flowers from friends and families. They loved their sweet little boy already. For Lucy, 'The one thing he wasn't was a disappointment. He was such a blessing.'

But being at home was hard. She persevered with breastfeeding but Charlie still couldn't suck. One weekend they stopped using the bottles and just breastfed. Then they noticed some pink residue in the nappy. The health visitor came and said Charlie was dehydrated and not feeding at all. They went back to the bottles, with Lucy expressing. Maybe, they thought, he would breastfeed later, when he was stronger.

A syndrome called ...

The appointments continued. Six weeks later a geneticist took a detailed case history and told them that Charlie had a syndrome called Möbius and that he would not have facial expression. Talipes had been part of it. They were devastated. Lucy now understood why Charlie would look at her so intently and why he couldn't feed. Yet, even at this time, his personality seemed so strong and his eyes gave her such a strong sense of connection that she believed he would be alright.

The geneticist gave David and Lucy an academic medical paper on the syndrome, warning them that it was a negative, clinical, portrayal of Möbius. Lucy is a university lecturer and David works for a large mental health charity. The doctor must have presumed the paper would allow them to understand Möbius but it contained stark medical photographs of babies; intellectually they might have read it with interest, but their intellects were not in charge. Their concerns were about Charlie's future; how would he cope? Would he walk? Would he be able to go to school? Would he fall in love?

Their paediatric consultant was supportive. They wanted to research the syndrome on the Internet and contact a support group. She warned them that the Internet is not regulated and might have information and experiences not relevant to Charlie. True enough, their initial soundings were very depressing, with reports of Möbius children confined to wheelchairs and having severe learning disabilities. They soon realized how rare Möbius is and that they were unlikely to find help close by. Their web search led them to the Möbius group in the United States and from that they drew strength from positive, happy, portrayals of children with the condition and stories of how valued these children with Möbius are. The support group sent a leaflet with a description and a photo of a child with Möbius, together with basic facts of Möbius and its characteristics. Not only was this reassuring; unlike the medical paper, the support group's literature had a human dimension.[2]

In parallel with medical visits, life continued. Charlie was a small baby, and compared with Hugh he did not move around much. In fact he spent much of his time just lying on his back. He would sleep, ask for food and then sleep again. 'He didn't demand our attention much, in part because he couldn't make good eye contact and smile.'

Feeding remained an issue and they spent a lot of time squeezing bottles, expressing and feeding. Sometimes, after a long feed, he would vomit and the whole thing had to be repeated. Fortunately, they had some high energy milk and at 12 weeks he started taking solids. He was able to swallow them much better and quickly he thrived and, at last, grew.

The stream of appointments continued. In the first eight months there were dozens, and this didn't even include the weekly plastering of his foot to straighten it. Yet Lucy remembers it as a lovely period. Surrounded by family and friends and support, they really enjoyed time with Charlie and, of course, Hugh, who had just started school.

Even before they were told of Möbius, Lucy knew that whilst a friend's little baby would smile in her sleep, Charlie did not. After diagnosis the penny dropped; he couldn't. Before that she had not realized exactly what it was he wasn't doing, so rapt with her new baby was she. Despite this she feels that her bonding with Charlie was similar to that with Hugh. But on the odd occasion, particularly when with other children, she noticed small things he did not do; one day she noticed that he didn't yawn in the same way. Even now, if a child smiles at her she thinks how clever, how amazing that is. Charlie's communications with her feel different. There were times when his lack of facial expression made life difficult. 'I didn't always know if he was OK – I couldn't tell.' Though they knew if he was happy or sad, from early on they were conscious that there were a whole range of emotions that they were missing. 'We would wonder if he was frustrated – whether there was a subtlety of emotion that he wanted to give us but could not.'

One day, at Woburn Safari Park, when he was around six months, they were looking at the penguins and Charlie went into peals of laughter. 'It was a wonderful moment to discover that he was amused by something – the laughter was a real signal of what was happening in his head.'[3]

At nine months Lucy's maternity leave came to an end and she returned to work part-time. Charlie started nursery two days a week.

They had briefed the nursery in advance about Möbius. Lucy's main concern was how they would know he was upset or happy, hungry, or needed his nappy changing. Yet, right from early on, the staff picked up the clues. They read whether his energy levels were high or low, what his body language was saying and even the tone of his voice. It was such a relief for David and Lucy that other people were able to figure him out. It worked the other way too; the nursery staff unwittingly confirmed to Lucy and David that they were interpreting their baby correctly too. But, more importantly perhaps, Charlie loved the nursery and loved playing and chatting with the other children.

Initially, Lucy thought that she should explain to people why Charlie looked different, both to help him and to save others from embarrassment and awkwardness. Gradually, though, she learnt to let people take him as he is and only chip in as necessary. At the preschool group she would find herself worrying what people thought, but sometimes she overanticipated and was almost too protective. Recently he was queuing up to go on the slide. Being a little slower and less agile than other children, another little child knocked him over. Lucy's first reaction was to step in and rescue him. Just then Charlie picked himself up, elbowed the other child out of his way and calmly carried on with his turn.

As time passed, Charlie's mobility became of more concern. Other children his age were learning to walk whilst he remained slower and unsteady. His balance was poor, too, resourceful though he was. Once, in the garden, he could not go down a step upright: he decided to sit down and slide down on his bottom. But what is charming at one age may not be so easy later. When he was 18 months old, Charlie had an operation on his foot, which was partially effective but still leaves him with problems in walking and balance. Lucy sometimes wonders how mobile he will be and how he will cope in the playground.

Not so different

Much of their early efforts were spent on Charlie's everyday requirements as a baby with Möbius – drinking and eating, making sure he could see and hear, so that it was only in the spring, when he was over a year old, that they started to think about finding out more about the longer term effects of Möbius. They discovered a conference in Dallas for children and adults and their families with Möbius. The timing seemed right to go, though they had no idea what they were going to. They had never met anyone with Möbius.

Checking into the hotel, in front of them was an American family unpacking a huge vehicle, a typical family scene with a girl of 8 arguing with her brothers. Then both Lucy and David noticed that she did not have all her fingers. Only then did they notice she also had Möbius. It was the first time they had seen another child and yet initially they had not realized. Suddenly, as they booked in, they were surrounded by children and adults with Möbius. Though tired from the flight, they were reassured to see so many little children with Möbius playing and running around.

Next day they found that there were so many different kinds of Möbius faces. Some had had surgery, some had had therapy; some were quiet, others were more outgoing and extrovert – just like the rest of us. Sure, it was strange, at first, talking to someone who cannot mirror your expression in conversation, but they soon found ways round it.

One reason they had gone was to see older people with Möbius. They were frank about wondering what their own beautiful boy might look like in the future. What would it be like to go through life looking 'disfigured' and having people react to one's facial difference the whole time? How could he get people to see beyond the Möbius? And yet, after a little while, they did seem to be able to see the person, with Möbius only a part of who they were. Meeting adults with normal lives and a jumble of jobs, families, partners, pets, friends, and hobbies was so important. Mostly though, they loved seeing all the children playing together; boys and girls with Möbius, toddlers and siblings, brothers and sisters all playing along together: playing football, dancing at the karaoke, playing Twister. 'It was really emotional watching Charlie play with other children who look like him. He's not so different.'

They returned from the States more confident. As Lucy says, 'It is so diverse. There is no one Möbius, each had varied involvement both mentally and physically. In coping we had to figure out what works for us.' At the conference they had had difficulties in understanding some people with Möbius, since without lip movement and often with tongue and jaw problems, some speech can be very difficult. Their next challenge was to see that Charlie had good speech therapy.

Some time ago, Lucy realized that a child with Möbius is still a child. Charlie was naughty and she told him off. She had this wonderful realization that as well as being their precious son he is still able to be naughty, just like any other child.[4]

Hugh has always been protective of his younger brother. Sometimes it has been difficult for him, especially with Charlie being treated as the fragile one. It has been particularly hard for Hugh to explain to his friends about Charlie. Hugh has even sometimes felt different and less special because he doesn't have Möbius. But as soon as another child came to peer into the pram then he would become incredibly protective. It was hard for Hugh since he didn't always get responses back from Charlie like he did from other children at school. But now Charlie has started to talk he has become much more interesting to Hugh and they play much more together.

Once Charlie started talking, it became easier to know what he was feeling. Not necessarily by his language, for babies do not start by saying how they feel, but in his tone of voice, gesture, posture, and whole physical demeanour. To see this is to realize how the actual words convey only a part of the meaning. This was a huge leap forward, allowing Lucy and David to demand more from Charlie, stimulating him and engaging him. They were so excited that he could answer back.

Charlie reached his second birthday. David and Lucy have had an amazing journey from their first difficulties with conception to becoming experts in Möbius; *their* Möbius in *their* Charlie. They know no more about the future than any of us, but curiously have come to consider Möbius less and less. As Lucy said:

> 'We are so busy that Möbius has become such a small thing in our everyday lives. He remains our wonderful boy. We take one step at a time and just hope we have the tools to make his future OK.'

Still my baby

Not for a moment does one have the impression that Lucy and David doubt the joy of Charlie's arrival. Another parent of a Möbius child agreed.

'I was 39 and had waited so long for this. The name [of the syndrome] was not important, he was my much-loved baby. I talked to him all the time; the nurses and doctors hid behind the curtains checking, listening, and then went away satisfied. No smile – he was still my baby; some brain damage, still my baby.[5] They told me that his lack of a smile might lead to problems with bonding. I never could understand that crap.'

But not all parents find it so easy.

Sian's father was in the army and she was born during a posting in Germany. Living in a camp, away from many old friends and family, her mother, Mary, struggled, not least because they were avoided by the other mums and families; her only visitors came to see the 'freak baby'. Worse, the doctors told her Sian would be 'a vegetable'.

Mary grieved for the loss of the child she had wanted. Looking back, if there had been a prenatal test she would have considered termination. She found it so difficult that Sian could not show any facial response to what was going on around her, whether a noise, or a light or to her – not a smile, not a grimace, not one of the funny faces most babies make. It was frustrating, lonely – and maddening; this little thing she loved so much didn't respond. At times she wanted to hit her just to get something back. How could you know if she was happy, sad, uncomfortable, or bored? How was she to know what her baby was thinking or feeling? How could she care for her and love her if she couldn't read her?

As she grew so Sian proved the doctors wrong. She crawled and laughed and showed her family that she wasn't a vegetable after all. When they were finally given the diagnosis of Möbius, when Sian was around three, it came as a relief. Möbius syndrome was a fairly minor thing compared with what they feared might be wrong.

A blooming buzzing confusion?

William James [1890] famously described an infant's initial experience of the world as being a 'blooming, buzzing confusion'. This underpins what has been a traditional view; that babies learn about their bodies, and about the world, over their first months and years, and that the contents of their consciousness are formed by learning from their sensory experience and their exploratory movements. We start with what Stephen Pinker [2002] has called 'the blank slate'. Merleau-Ponty [1964b] suggested that experience is derived from internal sensory experience alone for the first few months and that, gradually, as the senses develop, so external experience becomes increasingly ordered and understood. He also suggested that control of movement was linked with sensory learning; without postural control of the head and eyes to see the world, and exploratory movements through the world, either literally of the body or via eye movements, then perceptual experience would be impoverished.

Such a view led Piaget to suggest that imitation in infants of another person's movements, using parts of the body invisible to that infant, was not possible until that infant had a relatively mature motor schema, or set of motor programmes or plans [Piaget, 1962]. These arguments were particularly directed towards facial movement. This was because, as Merleau-Ponty suggested, for a baby to imitate the facial expression of the other, she (or he) would have to have seen the other's facial expression and then translate this into a motor language, in order to reproduce that expression, even though she could not see her own face (though it could be felt through internal proprioceptive feedback).

These ideas about motor development and imitation were dominant until a series of famous experiments by Meltzoff and Moore beginning in 1977 [Meltzoff and Moore, 1977]. They showed that newborn infants can imitate facial expressions within one hour of birth, and subsequently others have found examples of babies able to do this within a few minutes of birth, for 'big' facial gestures such as a wide open mouth or tongue protrusion. Meltzoff and Moore also showed that babies a little older, at 16 to 21 days, also had a short memory of what facial expression to imitate too.

This work negated previous ideas about the gradual development of motor control of the body, and sensory experience of the world, at least in relation to others. A newly born infant could imitate, could see others move and move herself similarly, without having to see that movement in herself. Some motor programmes or schema, at least, were not a result of training but were innate.[6]

The other aspect of significance is what Meltzoff and Moore termed intermodality; the infant recognizes the seen face of the other visually and uses a motor programme to imitate it. In addition, as Gallagher

[2005] has argued, for success in this there must also be a mature form of performance awareness; the infant must have some feedback to guide the process. All these are far from the limited performances of Merleau-Ponty and Piaget, and from James' buzzing confusion.

Yet in all the excitement these observations have generated in psychology and philosophy, there has been less attention directed towards why these intermodal programmes are actually present so soon after birth.

When I first became interested in the experience of Möbius syndrome, I interviewed several adults with the condition, and parents of children. I attuned myself as best I could to the prosody, speech, and gesture, and the way people with Möbius thought about themselves. Then I went to a meeting of the UK Moebius Support Group and there I first saw a young baby with the condition, being wonderfully and lovingly looked after by his young parents. Nothing I had seen had prepared me to see this young baby with Möbius.

Without language, without gesture, and without much eye movement the baby lay there, with a few sounds and limited arm movements, but otherwise with nothing with which to communicate. A baby can cry, gurgle, and chuckle, expressing its needs for food or for a nappy change. But what is crucial for any baby's survival is not only to have these basic needs satisfied. It needs to build up interpersonal relatedness with its parents. For this, facial expressions seem crucial, for before gesture and before speech and language, the face is arguably the most important channel for a baby to show her parents that there is someone home. More, by mimicking facial expressions between each other, child and parent share and exchange affective, emotional embodied expressions and feelings, through vision, through the face, right at the beginning. Every mother and father sees their young baby and beams a big smile across, imploring its return. Before I saw that baby with Möbius I could not have imagined the force with which this became evident. Lovers gaze into each other's faces (their visible souls) endlessly during courtship and attraction can be – initially – a face thing as much as anything, but perhaps even above this, the face is most important in those early days when a baby shows itself to its parents.

One can, therefore, understand Mary's frustration about Sian. Though there are stories of parents who reject their offspring, many – most? – parents of children with Möbius transcend this lack of returned and reinforced emotional communication through face in other ways, through voice and hugs and, as in the baby at the Support Group, watching them do this was very moving. For Vicki McCarrell, who was the prime mover in the wonderful US Moebius Syndrome Foundation, the birth of her son, Sean, was a joyful celebration, with his Möbius but a part.

'He looked into my eyes. I had no clue that babies move their faces; he moved his arms and legs, so? I talked to him all the time.' Weeks later she went round to a friend's house to see her baby and was slightly surprised. 'I saw this friend's baby doing all these things with his face and I thought "Ugh, that's too much." My friend just smiled and said that is what they are supposed to do.'

Chapter 3

Balancing acts

At the beginning is the shock; with feeding, with the impairments like talipes, and with the name (assuming that is met early on). Then there is the explaining, to one's parents, friends and relatives and then, later, to schoolteachers and new friends, and the endless visits to specialists and support workers of various kinds. Life is busy enough for parents with a newborn; it is busier still for those with a son or daughter with Möbius as they balance work and their own needs, support their child with Möbius and yet avoid disrupting the life of the new baby's brothers or sisters.

A busy start

Gemma is 12 and lives with her parents, Ken and Diana, her younger brother, Rob, and their chocolate Labrador, Cadbury. She also has four grown-up half-brothers and sisters. At school she likes English and art, dancing, and music. Her other great interests are Egyptology and Cleopatra, and she spent one summer teaching herself Japanese. Gemma is quite bright.

She was born at night, after an exhausting delivery, a failed induction and an emergency Caesarean section. Her parents were told that they had, 'A lovely little daughter, very beautiful, but with a bit of a short jaw. She resembles a successful actress ...' Feeding problems led her to the special care baby unit. By next morning she had had a brain scan and other tests, and Gemma's parents were given a provisional diagnosis of Möbius syndrome. The doctors explained about the facial paralysis, that her eye movements were also paralysed and that she might also need speech therapy. The next day the regional neurologist and eye specialist saw her and a multidisciplinary support team was arranged. Gemma's parents were amazed by the hospital team's speed and thoroughness.

She couldn't close her lips around the teat, or suck, so Mum's expressed milk was put in a syringe with a large teat. Diana held the syringe between her thumb and her index finger, Gemma's cheeks between middle and ring finger, and squeezed. It was a long slow process taking many hours each day; any remaining milk was put down a nasogastric tube.

After two weeks, Mum was discharged home. Gemma was kept in a further week because of concerns about her weight gain. Once home she had a near-continuous round of feeding and sleeping, with the former almost as long as the latter. Two weeks later they had their first review with their paediatrician; from then on began a round of doctor's trips, hospital visits and check-ups which has lasted, so far, 12 years.

A doctor friend found Ken and Diana articles about the syndrome, one of which mentioned the Smile Surgery conducted by Dr Zucker in Toronto. They contacted him when Gemma was still only a few weeks old. Diana mentioned this to their paediatrician who referred them to a plastic surgeon. He examined Gemma and found a partial cleft palate. This helped explain why feeding was quite so difficult and why food came back down her nose. Gemma would almost certainly also have glue ear and need grommets.[1] Because of the risk of airway collapse they needed to minimize the number of anaesthetics and they decided to do these all together. Meanwhile a mild neural hearing loss had been found by audiologists; Gemma would require hearing aids. Her small jaw also made anaesthesia more difficult.[2] She would need to be cared for in intensive care for 24 hours after surgery.

'I cannot describe handing over your 11-month-old baby outside the operating theatre and watching her go off to sleep. Not having any control over your baby is absolutely awful.'

Diana and Ken paced the corridors, walked the hospital grounds, sat in the ward, and jumped every time the phone went. The procedure was, in the end, straightforward and Gemma's feeding improved hugely. But at about the same time she began to develop squints. Initially she was given glasses, but at 23 months both squints were successfully corrected.[3]

As she grew her speech became increasingly challenging. Whilst her comprehension and language development was average or above, she found the production of sound difficult.[4] At a special-needs nursery they had help from a speech therapist twice a week, soon moving to one-to-one sessions on sound production. There were so many sounds she was unable to make; without lip movement: b, c, d, f, g, m, n, j, p, q, t, v x, z – at least half of the alphabet – were a trial. Another operation, a pharingoplasty, to close the pharynx a little, allowed her to add the g and k sounds to her repertoire.[5]

Apart from the odd gap, Gemma has been able to produce speech for the last ten years; it is time consuming and slow but they are making progress. Her Mum and Dad understand her most of the time, but it can be more difficult for others. After a while it is possible to 'tune in' but this is more difficult because it is not possible to lip-read Gemma, and because her face does not reveal the signals that other faces do.[6] She is now working on slowing down speech by focusing on exhalation; extending the amount of air in one breath allows her to speak more clearly. As she becomes more and more independent, comprehensible speech is of increasing importance.

Despite the lack of facial expression, Mum could always tell Gemma's needs from her tone of voice. Whether she was hungry, tired, or cross, Diana recognized different tones and pitches. From her reading and contact with the support group, Mum was also aware that whilst Gemma was unable to make facial expressions herself, it was most important that she was exposed to the whole range of expressions by her parents and siblings. Early on, Diana developed an exaggerated form of body language to convey emotional meaning to Gemma. If angry, she would place her hands on her hips to emphasize her message and she encouraged Gemma to do the same. She would also mimic her daughter to reinforce her use of expression, by a shake of her head or waggle of her finger, etc.

> 'Can we find another way around this, what can we do instead? There was no "can't". You might not do something this way but you find another. There are so many different ways to convey emotion – you use your eyes, the sound of your voice, your body.'

But, on her own, Diana would spend hours in front of the mirror, trying to imagine what it would be like to have no facial expression, trying to think of any gestures that might help. Above all, she wanted to understand what Gemma might be feeling.

The badge

Diana registered Gemma for school and discussed Möbius with the Head. The school was welcoming and assured her that they would find a way to cope. Diana was particularly concerned about teasing. Gemma started nursery with her next-door neighbour. Even though Gemma struggled to express herself, she still took part in everything. The teachers, prepared by an adviser for the hearing impaired, gradually tuned into her speech. As her fine movements were still weak, she found drawing and writing hard but otherwise she developed well.

One day, when she was in infant school, she returned home despondent. The children had been told that the following week was National Smile Week. 'I haven't got a smile,' she told her mother. 'Yes you have. You've got your inside smile,' replied Diana, 'But they can't see it …'

Mum had an idea. They made Gemma a smile badge she could wear on her dress. If she did not want to smile she could pull her cardigan over it. The School Head suggested that Gemma got up in assembly to talk about her special smile. They gave the children a little explanation, and Gemma wore her smile during National Smile Week.[7]

The next big hurdle was at eight, when the children were placed in sets for reading and maths. As a bright child, she was placed in the top set. Gemma moved up with two other friends to a class with another ten girls and six boys she did not know well. It took her longer to settle than the other children, but with assistance from the Head and her team, a special needs adviser, a speech therapist, and a teacher for the hearing impaired, she coped well. Mum kept an active eye on everything from home.

In one test, Gemma did not do as well as expected. There was a meeting between school and Mum to identify the problem. The exercise had involved listening to the teacher, and then marking the answer in the correct space in a grid. Gemma had not been able to do this – her answers were out of sync. It turned out that she was unable to move her eyes and head to focus on the grid and move her head back down to mark in her answers on the exam paper in the given time. Gemma finds maths particularly difficult, because she cannot always see points on graphs. Her lack of balance, poor sight, and reduced sensory awareness make playing ball games tough, too. Jumping, throwing and looking at a ball, then judging distance, speed, and depth are all too much.

As Gemma grew older she began to notice that people would look at her differently and sometimes stare. She was upset and did not know how to respond. She wanted to know why she couldn't smile. As a family, they talked about Möbius and what it meant. In the end, though, there are only so many words.

Throughout her life, she has needed regular hospital monitoring and check-ups. Diana is doing everything to ensure that this all happens in the holidays, though this does mean that holidays can become rather hospital focused. They also have to fit it in around her brother and the rest of normal family life.

> 'She is doing so well academically and we don't want her to miss out. She is bound to have to work a little bit harder than other children to maintain her level and I just didn't want to complicate things by making it even harder.'

Soon after Gemma was born they went to their first Möbius Support Group conference:

> 'At first it was quite nerve-racking, and very emotional. There was so much information visually and verbally. Then we saw kids with Möbius running around, talking, doing this, playing, and we thought, "She'll be fine." There were just so many different strains and it took a while to assimilate. It's not that you are comparing but you just have to absorb and process.
>
> 'There is no one else who understands exactly. It is rare – you need to know there are other people out there, people who Gemma can talk and relate to. There are also so many different variants on the theme.'

They were helped by a couple of other families whose children have hearing problems. Their advice and information was invaluable and they also found out where the specialists were. By the second conference, they were more able to select what information and advice was relevant for them.

> 'You have had time to take things in. You are aware you don't want to upset every one but at the same time you are looking for the information which will help you. Every parent has a different agenda and a different take.'

Diana remembers the first time Gemma saw that there were other children like her. 'It was like being part of a big family; nothing mattered, everything was easy.' As she grew up, other "Möbians" became more important; sharing what it was like to have a photograph taken, say at children's camp or ballet exams. In the early years, they shared the practicalities and what therapies might be useful. As she has grown older, they have asked the group more questions about how others cope at school, how families deal with unkind comments from peers. Diana is especially concerned about Gemma in her teens.

Body brushing

They have tried a number of complementary techniques to try to improve Gemma's speech and function. They started with body brushing when Gemma was 2 years old; their expectations were not high. The theory behind this is that the body possesses a number of reflexes, which normally disappear at birth or shortly after. In Möbius children, for some reason, these reflexes are said not to disappear and it is believed that gentle body brushing corrects this. Möbius children are considered to require stimulation along the spine and down the sides, on the face area and around the hands. They invested much in this and were fortunate to have funding from their primary care centre.[8] For a while they achieved a partial blink; they also noted changes in her behavioural patterns, but several years on Gemma lost the blink.

The treatment remains controversial and unproven. Whilst the family appreciates that the doctors need scientific evidence on the therapy, 'As a parent you want your child to improve however they can and you will do whatever it takes.' They stopped when they felt that she was no longer progressing.

Next they used a neuromuscular stimulator they saw in a national newspaper. Gemma was hooked up to cables and electrodes connecting stimulation pads to her face at several places. Initially, aged four, she wore it for three hours a day, five days out of seven, or for longer. She would go to bed with it on. Now she uses it for 20 minutes with breaks from the routine. Gemma has made distinct improvements. Her bottom lip has come up and under the eyes has lifted; there are photos to show this.

They tried a biofeedback machine for a while. Gemma tried to make movements of her face, frowning, smiling, grimacing, trying whatever movement she could, and then saw a response through lights on an electrical box as the muscles worked. In this way, she has been able to train her face to do certain exercises. They have also tried acupuncture and other therapies with mixed results.

When Gemma was younger, Diana had researched smile surgery, and a decade later, they still haven't decided. They made an appointment at Mount Vernon Hospital where this was done. They have always viewed surgery as the last option; after all it involves two long operations, not without risk, and they wanted to explore other options first. They also thought that Gemma should choose herself, once she understood its implications. As yet they are not convinced.

'There are lots of issues to consider; scarring, whether your child will be happy with the result, after all you cannot recreate perfectly the smile. As parents we are not sure if we can make that choice.' Gemma pitched in too at this point, 'If you ask me if I want it, I have no idea.' It is difficult to know how she could have any idea at her age, or any age come to that.

Thank you for listening

At school, the sensory support service, speech therapist and adviser for the hearing impaired would visit once a term, or more often if necessary. Each time, they tested Gemma's hearing aid, ran a speech discrimination test and sat in on classes to check that she was sitting in an appropriate place. Later she was also helped with her visual impairment and her physical issues. She was poor at balancing, going up and down stairs, and judgement of depth, distance, and speed, especially in the playground. It was beautifully managed, though her parents were increasingly aware that she would soon go on to big school – secondary education where life would become more complicated with new teachers, new children and a different building. She would also need to pass an entrance exam, one of which involved a dreaded grid.

Early on, it had been decided that Gemma would not require a statement of her abilities and problems (a formal list of her problems introduced by the Local Educational Authority) since they did not want to codify her disability or label her. Retrospectively, they were not sure if this was for the best. They were unclear whether, as an academically bright child, she would have special educational needs. With the imminent move to a big school they reconsidered. During her last year at junior school, various assessments also suggested that she would benefit from a statement. As Diana suggested, 'Individually each of her particular needs is not a major problem but when they are added together the combination is very complicated.'

The application process was lengthy, involving visits by the community paediatrician, a report by an educational psychologist and consultations with teachers. Six months later the statement was granted. Gemma's statement details are focused around vision, hearing, and speech, physical problems, and ensuring integration based on medical grounds. For her family, the statement has been a reassuring tool. Her health and safety is paramount.

> 'What would happen if Gemma was badly positioned in the classroom so she could not sit in front of the blackboard? How would they manage with her copying slowly, not being able to hear, having to move her head from side to side to read, which slows her down, moving around the buildings when she might get lost, fall over, not see signs around the building, not see children running past. All these factors could have a detrimental affect to her learning to the best of her ability.'

Gemma passed her exams, and together they chose a school that had a friendly environment and was successful, without piling on the pressure. The teachers had also asked the right questions about Möbius when they went round. Once they accepted the place, an advisory teacher for hearing discussed Gemma's statement. Then Diana met the form teacher and deputy head to discuss Gemma's needs further.

There was a welcome afternoon for the children and some of the families organized a picnic in the summer holidays; a chance to meet before the first day. One major concern was how they were going to present Gemma and her Möbius to the rest of the class. Gemma wanted to be open from the beginning. They decided that the best way would be for Gemma to get up in front of the class and introduce herself. They prepared her the following brief, based on her experiences, those of her family and of other families in a similar situation they had met:

> 'Hello everyone. My name is Gemma and I live with my parents, my 9-year-old brother and my dog. I also have three grown-up brothers and one grown-up sister. I love dancing, listening to music, reading, and Egyptology.

'I was born with something called Möbius syndrome, which for me mainly causes facial nerve paralysis. This means that my face cannot express the emotions that I am feeling. For example, it can't form a smile when I am happy. However, even though I am not able to smile at you on the outside, you can be sure that I am smiling on the inside!

'I have a mild hearing loss so I wear hearing aids for some of my lessons and these allow me to hear everything clearly.

'My speech isn't always as clear as I would like it to be, so if you need me to repeat something I've said, please ask me.

'I hope you will agree that no two people are alike and it is our differences that cause every human being to be special. Thank you for listening.'

She also had a photocopy for each child in case they had not been able to understand all she had said. She enjoys school and is doing very well academically and is near the top of her class in some subjects. 'She hasn't had a bad day, we haven't looked back.'

There has only been one unpleasant incident – at a sports practice she was called nasty names by a boy. First, he started teasing her and then he called her, 'alien,' 'outsider,' saying, 'Oh look, the alien's trying to speak English, translate for me.' This was the only time she has experienced name-calling. The form teacher pointed out to the boy that he needed to think about what he was saying and the impact it might have on Gemma.

Friends and future

Gemma has four best friends, typical 12-year-olds, who love listening to music and dancing. Of course they also chatter, gossip, play, see each other at weekends, after school, have tea at each other's houses, and have sleepovers. But she is also different. While other friends have been able to go shopping on their own, Gemma has not. Diana explained,

'Crossing roads could be dangerous. Hearing aids amplify all sounds, including background, so walking around outside can be quite noisy. She might not always be able to determine where traffic comes from. If someone toots all of a sudden, she might go into a quick panic.'

Recently she has had orientation training from the Association for the Visually Impaired and she is learning the right way to cross the road. Another factor that complicates matters is judging distance, depth, and speed. Telling when an approaching car is actually going to pass by can be very difficult. How close is it? How fast is it going?

Being unable to move the eyes in the head makes such tasks more difficult and, when combined with the hearing impairment, makes street life tricky. The roadside kerb can be difficult to negotiate, and if she was lost she might ask someone to help her and they might not understand her speech. One of these problems might not hamper her, but summed together they are significant. Choking is another hazard. Should the family give the responsibility to the friend if she goes and has lunch out? Could they trust people's Heimlich expertise? If she wants to go the cinema, her parents take her and pick her up afterwards. If she wants to go shopping they take her to traffic-free zones, as they feel it is not fair to ask her friends to shoulder the responsibility.

Diana and Ken are trying to prepare Gemma for the next stage of life – her teenage years. Everything is done in small, manageable, bite-size targets. When shopping, Gemma now has to ask for what she wants, pays, and gets her change. Each is a small task, but in speech therapy terms huge; speaking to a complete stranger and carrying out a whole transaction is very difficult. Sometimes progress is slow.

Now 12, Gemma is still learning to live with Möbius. She does not like it and on bad days she is annoyed by it, especially her inability to smile and her frustration at not being able to speak clearly. Her main worries for the next years are boyfriends. She hopes they will be able to see her personality. She knows she is at a different starting point from her schoolfriends. But she does have plans for her future, big plans, though simple ones. 'To be an award-winning author, become a millionaire, and buy lots of houses.'

Mum's hopes are lesser – perhaps.

'It is hard, but we want her to be happy in what she does, to be as secure as possible. We hope we have given her some of the tools to face the future. Ultimately, it's up to Gemma what she chooses to do. Sometimes it still seems an uphill struggle.

'We want to be sure we have accessed all the information and options and have investigated as many potential therapies as possible; anything that might make life easier. However, at the same time, it mustn't take over our lives; we need to balance it with the rest of family life. A child must have a childhood too.'

They are still seeking a balance that works for everyone in the family.

A litany of care

At a recent international meeting in Bethesda, there was a session on the treatment needs for those with Möbius. These ended up as a long list, stretching through childhood and beyond. Initially, there was help with feeding and nutrition. Then the child might need ophthalmological surgery for correction of squint, eyelid surgery to protect the cornea, facial surgery for smile surgery, and static procedures for facial droop. Tear ducts may also not be functioning normally and need surgery. Dental visits were required since with a small, inelastic oral orifice and subsequent dry mouth dental caries was more frequent. Young children with Möbius also had reduced development of the dental enamel, and often an open bite, with the teeth not closing on each other, which could lead to the tongue thrusting forwards to make a seal when swallowing. Adults with Möbius often use their tongue as a bottom lip when drinking. They also had gum disease, dental crowding, abnormal-shaped teeth and missing teeth, together with chewing problems, tongue underdevelopment, soft palate, and palate problems, all of which required regular assessment and treatment. Not surprisingly, some children become more than reluctant to have frequent visits to the dentist. This may be exacerbated by their being especially sensitive to touch round the mouth. Major surgery may also be needed to correct club foot, which may involve an Achilles-tendon lengthening, and release of tendons and ligaments in the foot to allow it more flexibility. The aim is for one operation but sometimes several are needed – one person with Möbius has had ten operations on her feet thus far. Operations may also be necessary for palatal and pharyngeal problems as they were in Gemma.

In addition to surgery, there is also a long-term and time-consuming need for speech therapy. Sara Rosenfeld-Johnson, who has extensive experience of helping children with Möbius, finds that each person is different, making it difficult to generalize.[9] Sometimes a lack of good use may arise from a reduced awareness of what the mouth and tongue are doing. She can also find reduced oral sensitivity to touch but, paradoxically, some heightened distress when aware of touch too.

Normally, we play with our faces, touching it, moving it, speaking, and exploring the mouth with the tongue. We spend large amounts of time just touching the face with the hand, stroking, picking, and scratching. The face is a large part of our sentient body. Without movement of the face, children with Möbius don't tend to do this. It is as if the face is a lesser part of their body image, their perceptual embodied self.[10]

Speech therapists spend time making children with Möbius more aware of their mouths and the position of their tongues using a variety of sensory stimuli, including a small gentle vibrator with a soft ned. Sara Rosenfeld-Johnson teaches children how to feel a bubble on the lips, 'the bubble kiss' and how to chew on the back teeth and try to close the mouth as best they can. She introduces exercises for the lips, with straws and horn blowing, and graduates to giving puree to eat or slurp. It is very difficult to swallow with an open mouth and for that reason children with Möbius sometimes put their heads back to swallow. She tries to improve this. Her approach is that the mechanisms of speech and eating are similar and seeks to add to whatever function is present.

Traditional speech therapy is, of course, also needed, since the lips are used for many sounds including closing for 'm', 'b', and 'p', rounding for 'sh', 'ch', and 'j', and in other ways for vowels, such as the rounded lip 'oo' and retracted lips 'ee', etc. It is also necessary to ask children with Möbius to slow down in order to be understood more clearly. In parallel with speech therapy are assessments and treatment of hearing loss. There can also be clumsiness and poor balance, leading to difficulties with walking, stairs, kerbs, and a myriad of daily tasks, let alone with games. All have to be recognized and assisted where possible.

Children also need longitudinal educational assessment and developmental monitoring, and intervention if indicated, and support for the family or caregiver. In a careful analysis of behaviour in young Möbius children, and offering a tribute to their care, Briegel et al. [2007] found little increased problems in a group of 22 preschoolers in Germany but that there was evidence of higher levels of stress in their parents and primary caregivers, compared with a control population, (though not compared with others looking after mentally or physically handicapped children).

The aim in giving such a list – as painlessly as possible – is to show just how much medical care, as well as educational supervision and awareness, is required to allow a young person with Möbius to reach his or her potential. For the child herself it requires a continuing, daily level of effort and concentration that is difficult to imagine. Like many with various disabilities and impairments, the young Möbian has to try so much harder than her unimpaired friends just to get by, let alone to excel; arguably to get by is to excel. Gemma's achievements, despite poor hearing and speech, limited eye movement and poor coordination, are noteworthy in themselves, though no doubt she would just say she is getting on as best she can. Her parents might say the same about their role, judging the various medical and other interventions needed and preparing the way for Gemma at her schools, as well as giving her and her brother as normal a childhood as possible.

Key skills for the disabled

It was crucial that Gemma was in a mainstream school and, given all her medical problems and the time she has had to devote to the various treatments and therapies, it must have been a huge help that she is bright and at an enlightened school. Not all are as fortunate.

Jimmy, a university graduate, was born with Möbius, squints, club feet and only a thumb and little finger on each hand. As a young child, he was given speech therapy; he was mainly interested in cars and his first word was 'Renault'. Despite surgery, his club feet meant that he couldn't move around like the other children, so joining in was difficult. He sulked and learnt to play on his own. At 6, he was sent to a special school where he learnt, 'key skills for the disabled, painting and basket weaving.' Having an unusual condition was a problem. 'If you saw someone in a wheelchair, you would just think, "Oh, he's in a wheelchair." You wouldn't ask why. You would just take it at face value.'

In his teens, as part of his county's 'rationalization' of special schools, he was sent to the local comprehensive, with the laudable aim of integrating children with disabilities into normal schools. On his first day, he was assaulted by the school bully. Despite a special support worker, the bullying continued. Other children called him names, left him out of their groups, wouldn't let him play football. One girl singled him out, turning people against him, making his life very unpleasant. Other children seemed to think he was getting preferential treatment. The school did not intervene.

Lessons were little better. Excluded from mainstream schooling for years, he was way behind and placed in the lowest set for all subjects. The others came from a variety of backgrounds, petty criminals, those who had been sexually abused – none was academic. He left school with some minor qualifications only. It was only then, aged 16, that he decided he wanted an education and took himself off to a college for disabled people.

Surrounded once more by others with disabilities, he found friends and enjoyment in learning. He passed five GCSEs and then moved on to the local college and studied for his A levels. After this, like many young people, he was unsure what he wanted to do. He decided to do a course in journalism, discovered the student life and then went off to university, along the way seizing chances to study aboard. For Jim the biggest hiccough was mainstream schooling, though that reflected the school and his peers rather than the idea itself.

Mirrors

Gemma, in common with many young Möbians, would spend hours looking in the mirror, trying to get her lips to close, willing them to and maybe coaxing them together with her hands. She wanted a normal-looking, normally working mouth. At other times her mother would gaze into the mirror trying to imagine what it might be like to be Gemma, inside the facial immobility, inside the eye problems and the reduced hearing, poor speech and clumsiness, inside her Möbius. Mother and daughter were mirroring each other, one trying to find a way out of Möbius to a normal existence, the other trying to imagine what it must be to be inside, and inside as a child.

The rest of this book will largely be concerned with approaching this question, by asking adults with Möbius about their experiences. Many of these narratives will focus on the present, but before this, in the next chapter, Celia gives her thoughts on childhood. Now in her early fifties, her recall of what happened and what she was feeling then is amazing.

One problem with Möbius is its congenital nature; people with it have known no other world. A few years ago, I was interested in how people who are deaf (the community profoundly impaired in hearing from birth) differentiated the use of the face during sign language from our usual use of the face for emotional expression and communication. A colleague, Bencie Woll, very kindly arranged a seminar with several deaf people to explore these ideas. I outlined my questions and rationale and then soon realized a problem. For the deaf, this was a non-question. Facial and linguistic uses of the face were clearly and obviously different; why could I not see? I went away feeling I had wasted people's time and tried to understand where I might have gone wrong. I slowly realized that the deaf, who had known no other existence, may have found it difficult to dissect the two uses of the face. Maybe someone who had become deaf as an adult, those who the deaf call the 'hearing without sound', might have been able to answer my questions. Maybe, because they had had a change in their situation, they would have been able to realize the difficulty I had. It is those who have known profound change who might have had the insights I sought. This was certainly the case in those who lose their sight as an adult; they are often able to reflect on the very different worlds with and without sight that someone blind from birth might not.[11]

There is likely to be a similar difference between those with congenital facial disfigurement and those in whom disfigurement is acquired after burns or cancer as an adult. In the latter, one's personality and interests have been formed, though these may need to be re-formed and redefined after the problem. In contrast, those with Möbius and other congenital visible differences have known no being independent of their condition. It is all the more remarkable that Celia, who we now read about, has been able to reflect as she does, since her world has always been that of Möbius.

Chapter 4

Cartesian children

Memories

'The first thing I remember is lying on an operating table when I was about 3, with a horrible gas mask coming down. I remember a long, long Nightingale ward. I thought the nurses were really stupid because I had a nil-by-mouth notice and they gave me a sandwich. I knew I should not eat. The op had to be delayed.'

Since Celia, like others with Möbius, could neither close her eyes or move them, she had no option but to watch the mask, and the rest of the scene, until she was unconscious. Her operation was for talipes, which was making it difficult for her to put her feet down on the floor. By then she had already had several other operations.

'Shall I show you my special shoes?' She got up, went to her writing cabinet and brought out a pair of exquisite little boots she had kept; as a baby she had worn them for months. They had a metal bar between them to try to keep her foot from pointing down. She also showed me a large syringe, which had been used to feed her. She was a big baby because, 'They did not know when to stop feeding me.' Her early years were hospital and doctors, home and school.

'I did not do ballet, horse riding, etc., I did hospitals and operations. I had the eye doctor and the foot doctor and a speech therapist, who I don't remember, and a face doctor.'

She was never aware of not seeing before these ops but then, as she says, she cannot see well even now.

'My limitations were a fact of life. Not being able to see the blackboard, or not being able to see someone over there. I have, or had, a squint and astigmatism. The shape of the Möbius eye is also different and I cannot move the eyes or move the head so easily, my muscles being not so well developed. Crossing a road is still difficult. I cannot judge when a car over there is going to get to me. I cannot measure distance and moving, the velocity or whatever is out. As a child I could never catch a ball.'

As well as having the talipes, her feet were also painful. She never told anyone.

> 'No one asked. When I was 7, I stopped walking because the feet were so bad and I had to go to school in a wheelchair. I don't remember learning to walk. After some surgery I could walk but I never told anyone I was in pain. People don't ask little children. I always remember that as an adult I have had pain, but I don't remember pain as a child.'[1]

The myriad of conditions – feet, mouth, eyes, skin (and other ailments too) – and the countless visits to doctors and therapists had an unusual effect on the way Celia viewed herself.

> 'I never thought I was a person; I used to think I was a collection of bits. I thought I had all these different doctors to look after all the different bits. At half term, other children would go off camping or on swimming courses: I would see the doctors; this one, then that one. "Celia" was not there; that was a name people called the collection of bits.
>
> 'I did not like my feet; I liked my spirit because I was strong as a child. I liked my brain; I knew I had a brain. I loved reading and read very early on. I liked that bit. I could think and dream and imagine. I had an IQ test, which was very high. I was bright, so I didn't worry about the rest. Even though I was a collection of bits I always knew there was something strong inside that I had a mental dialogue with, but it was not the physical body; it was very separate from the physical.'

In his famous *Meditations*, Descartes, exploring certainty and the nature of identity, doubted his embodiment but could not conceive of existence without mind; this was where his famous dictum, 'I think, therefore I am,' originated. Celia here seems to be making a similar disjunction between herself as whole, thinking being and her imperfect body; Celia was a Cartesian child.[2] Not only this, she was unable to share anything of her internal, thinking world with others. Most talked down to her as she clocked everything and communicated little. She would have an internal dialogue with herself – with her Celia – in her thoughts and imagination. In contrast her speech with others was about matters of fact. No one seemed to know or care about her situation.

> 'At 5, the only talking I could do was big, about operations, say, to doctors; I could only talk to adults, about my bits, not about me. I could also talk about books. Adults were my friends, not children. I just could not do playing with the other kids.'

At her first school, a girl said, 'Oh, you can't close your mouth.' Celia thought, 'That's what it is. It was the missing link; I realized that all the missing things did connect, and before that I thought they all did different things. I knew my mouth was different, because I saw it in photos. I knew this but no one had said it in so many words. It was interesting.'

School wasn't bad in the early years though. Her lack of social skills prevented much of what school is about but she liked lessons and she liked to lose herself in the routine. Learning fed Celia – Celia the bright disembodied mind – like nothing else.

> 'I did not express emotion. I am not sure that I felt emotion, as a defined concept. At my birthday parties I did not get excited. There were people around excited, but I followed what they did.'

She was also preoccupied with whether people would come, so she could be 'one of them', even though she knew she wasn't.

> 'I don't think I was happy, or even had the concept of happiness, as a child. I was saddened by being in pain or having horrid things like a blood test. Sometimes I would cry but even that would almost be a delayed reaction. I would have been sad so long the tears would come as I did not know what to do.'

Occasionally tears would come as a way to show people how sad she was but this was often because she could not deal with a situation. Once, a 'helpful' mum at a birthday party told her to close her mouth when eating. She did not know what to say, since she knew already that the mother would not understand. So she cried so she could leave the situation and the party.

> 'At the time, I just endured it. I could not express my feelings. Sure, I saw children in the playground laughing, but I always related it back to the physical. I did not know about an emotional world. I thought it might be related to my legs.
>
> 'I knew that being happy was something I couldn't do. Everyone told me I couldn't smile. I never got excited at Christmas. I watched others being excited. I verbalized it but not in an emotional way. I knew things were not as they should have been, even though I did not know how they could have been different. I was the eternal happy-ending girl. Even though things were pretty grim, as a child you don't have a choice, you cannot just stop.[3] I did not realize I was unhappy, I just was.'

She loved boarding school stories, which were closer to her experience than those of her contemporaries. In stories, there was always someone who lay in bed for weeks with pneumonia or TB; she had to lie in bed a lot too. From the happy endings, she developed the thought that it would be alright in the end. One girl at school had diabetes so they became friends, both knowing the sorrows of difference, though they never discussed their problems. Joining in with the others, in contrast, was always difficult.

> 'Doing something, like skipping in the playground, I was always at the end holding the rope not skipping. But at least then I joined in a game. I was actually important, because no one else wanted to be at the end. I felt part of the group; it was a warming, feel good sensation.
>
> 'Now, as an adult, I will say, "This is nice!" when I see something I like, just as you smile. Then, with adults, I would have a conversation but with children I was a bystander. Children had another language, a word language, a body language, a facial language. They run around and jump up and down and I could not do that because my legs did not work and because of my lack of balance.'

I suggested it must have been a bit like being in a foreign country, seeing the others sharing a communication she could never break into, as though she had mislaid the phrase book. She agreed.

> 'I was abroad once on a train with a friend speaking English and a man asked if he could join the conversation. He thanked us and said he had learnt English from the World Service but never spoken it before. As a child I just listened but never spoke their language. I witnessed it but never expressed or lived it. I thought I was strong inside, but the bits let me down.'

She would enjoy simple times, with her family especially, but even then the bits intruded. Looking forward to the theatre, or going on holiday, her body would often let her down and then she couldn't go at the last minute. She learnt early on that she could not rely on, or trust, her body. In fact, her body was as much or more of a problem as her face and her poor sight, and one of its worst parts was the pain she lived with with her feet, despite all the operations. It is still there.

> 'I live with pain all the time, in my feet whenever I walk ... I know it is there but if I told everyone everyday they'd get bored, (as I do with it).'

A smile?

The diagnosis of Möbius was not made until Celia was a toddler, around three. Having a diagnosis allowed her family to understand. For them, it meant that her collection of bits were part of a whole. But it meant far less to Celia. At that age she did not make any connection nor understand what it meant. Even later it was a hazy idea.

'At 5, it was about the mouth; I was not conscious of the facial expression thing. Even at ten, I just wanted my mouth to close and then everything would be OK. Everyone with Möbius spends time pushing their lips together. I did realize, however, that my face did look different and knew that this might explain people's behaviour, with them being kinder and more sympathetic to me. It was not just the face that looked different either, all of it seemed to.'

Aged ten, she saw a maxillofacial surgeon who arranged a masseter transfer to try to help her feeding and speech.[4] It was innovative at the time and she had lots of medical students coming to see her in hospital, as well as being filmed.

'Everyone from school made me cards; I had over 100. I felt very special – I knew I was special inside – and my wonderful headmistress called me Princess Celia and so she knew I was special too. I am not sure what the surgeons did, but I have scars under the cheek and inside. Masseter was the jaw-closing muscle; they connected it instead to under the mouth so it puckers in. It looks a little like smile surgery.'

She was in hospital several weeks and could not go to school there because they had measles. There was a little girl in isolation after a scald and no one visited her, even on her birthday. Celia's mother was there every day, having parked her other daughter and son with friends. The doctors also made her feel special too, and, to be fair, she was special having such surgery at this time for such a rare condition. 'Afterwards I had to learn to suck through a curly-wurly straw.' Straws are so hard for people with Möbius to use without cheek movement. She crushed it partially to make it easier to use. But she did end up with a sort of smile and improved lip closure. Afterwards she was able to chew without the food escaping, though the new movements have remained an effort.

'It is still not involuntary to use the "smile", many years later. I do it. I must have been told that it would be helpful as a smile. I did not work it out, so they must have told me. Everyone remembers the first bit of movement I had; we had to work at it. I had to do exercises. I think that was a pivotal moment for the family, the first time they had been able to create something in the face. It was not so much for me, though it was useful; it was more for the others. The early 1960s were an aesthetic time and concealing difference was important. It allowed them to feel I was more like them and that they had done something to help me.

'I don't use mine as a smile. I use it when I see people for the first time, since it is useful to them, but it is not good for me since I have to remember to do it. For me it is an echo. I have to stop speaking or drinking in order to do it. It is a voluntary action, very different to your use of the face.[5] But I recognize increasingly that it is useful for the listener to have reassurance and I have used it more for that over the last few years.

'It must have also helped with feeding; it was easier to chew, since the food did not all go into the cheeks. I used to be a real hoarder and since chewing was so difficult, I kept it in the cheeks. Without tongue mobility and no ability to shut the lips it was difficult.

'I missed loads at school and when I went back everyone commented. It became known as my little smile though it had no relation with emotion, which is what a smile is. It allowed a performance. Later on, aged 13, I was still stuck trying to close my lips so I had a slight broadening out of the top lip done by a plastic surgeon. That was for me. We also talked about a sling for my mouth, but the surgeon decided against it, so the compromise was the top lip. That was a slight let-down for me; it did not make my face like other people's.

'No one sat down and told me how the face works. It was all about the mouth and not about how the whole face works. Your forehead, for instance, tells me masses, but mine tells you nothing. I gradually became more and more aware that others' faces did things. It was not a revelatory moment, it was from when I was quite young, seven, eight, or so. I did not think, I saw.[6] People's faces were doing something; teachers are a good example, they are often demonstrative in front of the class and perform. It is very hard in any case when you can't see much anyway. So I saw this more from teachers than contemporaries. I related more to teachers.

'It made things easier, since you would know how they were feeling. I was conscious of people not knowing about me, what I was thinking and feeling. A person in my form was fairly moody. The teacher said when she was cross that it was because she had red hair. I was aware that people did not know with me, but then I did not know either; I did not have a clue.

'I did not know that I could tell people. The body is a transmitter of various clues. I thought the only way I could show people was the voice. Any non-verbal clues were divorced from me. I did not know they conveyed a message. This broadened the gap between them and me. The more I could see and read other people's faces the more they were different from mine. I also associated it with being patronized. I did not like my face and I did not think other people liked my face, so I shouldn't either. I never stared in the mirror because I did not like what I saw. I did not want people to look. I did not want to be noticed even before adolescence. I did not know what facial expression did and was for. I did not understand it showed feeling and expression.'[7]

Duncan – as a young boy[8]

It is possible that Celia's reflections on a time without happiness, indeed without emotion, are unique; perhaps others with Möbius are less affected. But perhaps, instead, it is her memories of childhood and her ability to find words to reflect which are rare, rather than the experience itself.

I went to talk with ten-year-old Duncan and his mother. Duncan, bored, soon left to play outside alone. His mother began,

'My other children had been precocious; smiling, sitting, standing earlier than most other children. With Duncan it was quite the reverse … there were odd things; for instance the other children recognized me when I went in the room – Duncan's never done that.

'Then, suddenly, I realized that he was no longer a baby and yet was still not doing things. By eight months, people were whispering that something was wrong. My other children had been smiling and crawling around by then but Duncan didn't do anything. He was a very cuddly baby but he never returned the smiles. The first time I really understood what was going on inside his head was one day when I was looking for a nappy pin for my youngest and he said, "Me get it," and he went and fetched it from the draw. He was 3 then. Up until then no one had known what intelligence Duncan might have.'

He had been completely passive, seeing and hearing, and yet unable to impose a sound or thought or emotion upon those around him. He went to a special school early and improved enormously with physiotherapy and speech therapy. He had a 1:1 helper for 25 hours a week, helping him with hand and speech problems. At school all he wanted was a wheelchair so that he could go abseiling down walls like the other kids.

He soon learnt that the Möbius was not only a handicap: sometimes he would bully smaller boys. Because he was such an innocent-appearing boy and did not show emotion, people were unaware of what he could do. No one could tell whether he was lying or not – you actually had to catch him.

'He just sits there like a little stuffed dummy – he doesn't touch his face as we do during gestures. We had to teach him to feel his face because he was dribbling.'

In place of the spontaneous and sometimes volcanic emotions children experience and display, and then learn to control, Duncan appeared calm and unemotional.

'Once, after his brothers had been unkind, he waited until they went out to play and then he went upstairs to their bedroom and smeared toothpaste all over the inside of their beds. We smelt something for a long time but it was only in the evening that we realized what he'd done. He really thinks about what he does and he never does the obvious thing. For instance, he hides things to torment people; one shoe for instance. He thinks about things far more before he does them than our other children. He's often off in his own little world working out what to do.

'He can sit up all night, till 3 or 4 o'clock in the morning and he'll pop down and eat something in the cupboard. We don't know what's going on in his head; he's too busy to sleep.'

Of course, with eyes that cannot be closed sleeping can be difficult. There is also evidence that sleep itself may be disturbed in Möbius (see Chapter 13). The highlights of a normal childhood seemed to pass Duncan by:

'I remember his fifth birthday party: he was sat in his high chair and went to sleep; it was just like another day for him. He didn't want to know, he didn't want to play. He doesn't really get excited on birthdays, even his own.

'It is difficult to know when he's having fun. When he comes home from school, we don't know how he's feeling, we have to ask him. Everything is questions and answers. He has always been a very placid child. He never really gets angry, never really appears upset.

'One thing, however, that clearly upset him is a lack of friends at school. He would come in from school and go upstairs to sulk and only re-emerge when he feels better.'

His mother continued,

'I wish I had taken more photographs. Because he never did anything and you usually take milestones, I never took them. He always sits back and listens and stores things for later; much more reflective. We always cuddle him but it's true that, probably because he's so thoughtful and reflective, our approach to him is less spontaneous. I used to cuddle him but he never really cuddled back. Now I still cuddle him because he's my baby but he just sits there saying, "I'm too old for this now, Mum."'

Clare

I had met Clare and her parents at a Möbius Support Group and asked if I could visit them in their home. She was in her early thirties; her parents were nearing retirement age. When we met again, I began by asking Clare about her childhood. Her mother replied,

'When she was born she couldn't suck. We tried everything, from small spoons to baby feeders, and in the end we used a soft teat. When she was eight months we took her to Great Ormond Street, where they made the diagnosis but didn't give us much indication what it would mean. Her father asked if she was backward and they said she might be a bit behind. She was slow in her milestones – she didn't speak really until she went to school and she went to an educationally subnormal school, (now called a school for those with learning difficulties). We don't think she should have gone to that school – she could have coped with the main-stream school but for her face – she'd have certainly coped because of her intellect.

'She's always been very highly strung. If she was sitting down or in a pram and I'd walk out of the room she'd scream. She screamed a lot. If I didn't take her with me everywhere, she'd scream; if I went upstairs she had to come with me – she went everywhere with me.

'We didn't have a night's sleep for four years; she used to scream and wake us up. Thinking back, I realize it was because she couldn't shut her eyes. She may have woken up and been frightened of the dark. Maybe if we'd had a small light in her room it may have been better. To wake up in the pitch black and be unable to see anything must have been terrifying.

'If she did not talk until she was 5 or so, I wondered what was going on in her mind. I imagine she thought a lot, I don't know. When I was in the room she followed me with her eyes and her head, of course, but as soon as I left the room she'd yell.'

They worked her into school gradually, initially in the morning then for a bit longer and then a whole day. They told her mother to leave her and Clare was fine. She did not have any screaming or tantrums. As her mother continued,

'School gave her something to do. Now she feels rather cheated because life has passed her by. She reads in church and she gives Communion. She could have done more. She sees her sisters getting on and she hasn't. She goes to a day centre just for something to do and they do various projects. Her friends are all older people, both in church and at the day centre.'

Clare was sitting next to me; though I was a little surprised by some of her mother's replies, Clare herself seemed almost relieved to have such matters aired. Then, in answer to a direct question, she started to speak.

'My first childhood memory is of having my teeth out at 3; a big black mask came over my face. Even now if somebody goes towards me I can't bear it.'

Her mother took it up again.

'In really stressed situations she'd lose control. She couldn't cope any more and would fall down, kicking out, spluttering, and shouting. Once, she ended up in casualty. She's had two EEGs to see whether these episodes are epileptic.'

Earlier that year, she had a severe episode, whilst her mother was in hospital. Previously she had been seen by a psychiatrist about her emotional outbursts. This time she walked round to the GP, apparently calmly, and asked to go to the local psychiatric hospital. Clare said,

'I remember, though I try and block it out of my mind. I know what's going on. I can't cope with assertive situations.'

She stopped, so I tried to help her out, suggesting that whereas some people might say something's awful, or even bloody awful, and then get angry, she might find it difficult to express emotions until they boil over; that she might go from being quiet and peaceful to a meltdown with little in between. She muttered that this was fair. Her mother suggested that this might be why priests have breakdowns, because they can't express emotion either. Clare spoke:

'I've always felt it difficult to express how I feel. I know it's only in the last couple of years that, say, at church, when I meet someone, I just say "I can't smile," and then it becomes easier. For 30 years or so I used to put it to the back of my mind. Now I'm beginning to be more aware of it.'

I wondered if she felt that the 'up and down' parts of her emotions were different from others.

'When I was young, I didn't know, I just accepted how I was. But it is happening now.'

I mentioned Celia saying that she had little emotional experience as a child.

'Yes, I feel that too. The spontaneity of feeling isn't as acute.'

I noted the present tense. She continued:

'I first met someone else with Möbius two years ago, at the meeting. It was wonderful. We sat in the hotel and we knew there was another one coming in and then another one and then another one and initially we were all a bit shy but by the next day we were talking to each other, swapping experiences. Because we all look the same its like one big family. I felt ... well, happy, really happy.'

I asked if she remembered getting excited at Christmas or birthdays. 'Not really.' Her mother continued:

'She was very quiet. For many years she would only go out with her sister or her parents. By the time Clare was 20, they'd stand at a bus stop. Sheila would get on the first bus and wait at the other end and Clare would get on the next one so that she would at least be on the bus on her own.'

I asked how she told someone she was sad:

'I don't – I can't. I think I've always been aware of such problems. At a wedding recently, the photographer kept saying, "Well smile!" to everyone and I had to say, "I can't smile." Maybe I couldn't have been so forthright a few years ago.'
'How do you tell someone when you're feeling good?'
'I don't.'
'Do you use body language much; might it help?'
'I do use it more, at church I recently leant over and touched someone. I may not have done that a few years ago. To wave back, even to someone I know, requires confidence and for a long time perhaps I wouldn't have done that.
'I very rarely went out when I was younger. Looking back, I wish I'd had more of an independent life. I really did enjoy being a care assistant. I enjoyed feeding the old people and I think they liked me 'cos they gave me an 18th birthday present, some china figures and a record.'

I returned to her attacks and asked if she had any warning.

'Yeah, I know for several minutes. Often I wake up feeling sad, or bad, and it's building up inside me, and I know its going to happen, and things progress. Though my mother doesn't realize it, I do know what I'm doing.
'I don't think people know how tense I am. It is very frustrating when no one knows how worked up I am. It's better now because I've found ways of telling them. At church, I used to read but I've stopped doing that – it made me too nervous. Now, I actually give the sacrament of Communion. I go to various places and actually stand there and do it.

A lot of people say they couldn't do it; they'd have to stand up in front of other people. It is quite daunting but I want to do it.'

'Do you feel that you observe life rather than take part in it? Might it be better if you could initiate things?'

'Yes. Exactly. Yes. That's it. Yes, that's very fair. If someone said, "Tell me what you want." I wouldn't know because I haven't sampled it.'

I began to talk more about the experiences of others with Möbius. I was aware that I might be leading her too much, but I also knew that if I did not discuss these things with her then she would surely never be aware of them. I also hoped that they might be useful for her. Others had said, I began, that being unable to express various emotions, not just happiness or sadness but all the different emotions, means that others sometimes think that people with Möbius can be passive. I suggested that if they were able to express emotion more, they would be able to experience it better themselves. Clare agreed. 'Yes, that's right. I haven't had those experiences. I just want to take part.'

Clare's sister came round and we chatted as best we could and I suggested some people who might be able to help. We kept in touch and some months later Clare moved out to her own flat. She would phone me every so often for support; we would talk late into the night. But then I heard she had moved back with her parents. Then, when I tried to meet them again they had moved and I could not trace them.

As we will see from the reflections of other adults, many with Möbius do have a reduced emotional life early on. They can be thought 'good' – passive and compliant – simply because they cannot impose themselves, their thoughts, and feelings, and character out in the world. Others can do this only in extremis, lacking the ability to learn how much emotion to express in a given context, leading them to express none, or too much both for them and for their carers.

The surgical smile

Celia mentions having surgery to give her better lip closure and how, as a by-product, she gained a 'smile' that was more for her family and others than for her. More recently, such surgery has become both more available and more refined. One of the pioneers, Ron Zucker from Toronto, has seen a number of people, mainly children, with Möbius as well as people with facial paralysis following other conditions, like tumour, Bell's palsy, and skull fracture [Manktelow *et al.*, 2006].

The technique involves taking a small amount of a muscle from the leg, with some of its nerve, and transplanting it to the face, where it is connected between the corners of the mouth and a muscle or fibrous band around the eye. The portion of nerve is connected to a small part of the nerve to the masseter muscle, which sits under the cheek in front of the ear and which normally closes the jaw. After three to four months, usually, the patient is instructed to practice smiling movements in front of a mirror, initially by making a biting movement, since that is what the nerve is wired to do. The patients then have to learn to create and control a 'smile', without any associated jaw closing. Then, over months, they try it out, initially with family and friends.

Though for Celia it has never become automatic and is always something she has to remember to do, for most of Zuker's sample, 89% of 27, smiling did become spontaneous some of the time. It became dissociated from biting all or most of the time in 69% of subjects. Of the four subjects who had surgery with congenital facial paralysis, which is not coexistent with Möbius, two were unilateral. All four could smile spontaneously, two all the time and two occasionally. Only one person out of 27, would not have the surgery done again.

Manktelow *et al.* discuss quite how a person might learn to 'smile' using a nerve wired to close the jaw. There was obviously an adaptation within the brain to enable this, even in adults, when such plasticity is less than in younger brains (they chose to study adults since they would be able to introspect better and communicate more). Each person had a long, intensive practice period sitting in front of a mirror. An important step was when they were able to contract the new muscle without biting, though how this was done is difficult to explain; 'It just happens.' They reported that patients were equally unable to explain quite how they introduce the smile into social situations. But, they suggested, an important point is when the person realizes that a smile will lead to the return of a smile by another person, that smiles are contagious and shared.[9]

Many people who have a facial nerve paralysis as an adult, say, due to Bell's palsy, complain of a numb face when they actually mean a paralysed one. The experience of not moving is felt as not feeling. It must be extraordinary to feel facial movement from the inside, for the first time, after smile surgery.

The mechanism by which a part of the brain learns to re-route in order to control the smile rather than jaw closing is unclear. In other such situations, such as after peripheral nerve injuries in the arm, when a nerve that is normally involved in breathing is reconnected to move the elbow, functioning imaging has shown that as the patient learns to move the arm, so the cortical brain area involved shifts from the respiratory to the arm. Manktelow *et al.* presume a similar mechanism here, though it is more difficult to show than the previous example since the 'jaw closing' and 'smile' areas are so close together. They do make the point, however, that because those who have had smile surgery with Möbius develop a spontaneous smile in some situations, they must have accessed a hard wired and congenital 'cortical smile area', or developed one as they learnt their new smiles.

Such arguments seem plausible, though in addition to investigating the motor cortical control of the smile, of interest are the felt experience of smiling in Möbius and its unconscious triggers. Do people with a new smile use it when happy, or when they meet people? Do they feel their face moving into a smile and does that add to the subjective experience of smiling and happiness? The nerves may join up and become automatic; but does the new smile join up to emotional experience, and if so does it extend the range of that experience?

Though these questions appear unanswered as yet; it is clear that for many smile surgery is very worthwhile. It can improve closure of the mouth and so improve eating, as well as allowing some facial animation, which is more socially acceptable; all of these help with self-confidence and social skills.

Interestingly, one person with Möbius describes how, when she feels emotion, she feels activity in the face, warmth, love, anger, etc. Even though no movement can be seen there is physical sensation there. The expression of emotion in the face does of course include autonomic activities like blushing and pupil dilatation as well as movement of the muscles of facial expression.

Junior Cartesians

In his book, *The God Delusion*, Richard Dawkins [2006] quotes Paul Bloom's suggestion that children have a natural tendency towards dualism, with an implicit distinction between body and mind:

> A dualist believes the mind is some kind of disembodied spirit that inhabits the body ... the idea that there is a me perched somewhere behind my eyes ... is deeply ingrained in me and in every human being.

As Dawkins suggests, there are few Cartesians amongst scientists (and few also amongst philosophers). But Celia's reflection goes beyond what most children think. We might think that our minds are where we are more than our body, but Celia felt she was a collection of bits which were defective and so not invested in and, importantly, that the real 'her', her mind and her self, could not communicate with others.

> 'Other children would go off camping or swimming; I would see the doctors ... "Celia" was not there; that was a name people called the collection of bits ... I did not like my feet; I liked my spirit. I liked my brain ... I could think and dream and imagine ... I always knew there was something strong inside that I had a mental dialogue with.'

There is an implication that the real Celia only talked with herself internally. The real Celia, for the first years after her development of reflexive awareness, was solitary, unable to express to others and locked within her defective, unreliable, Cartesian body by Möbius. Duncan might not have expressed himself thus as a child but one can imagine he might well be in a similar situation. How many similar Cartesian children with Möbius, and similar conditions, might there be?

I can remember being around 8, in the playground at school and seeing another boy who seemed to be more than just in the moment; he seemed to be thinking about something at one remove too, observing and analysing what was going on, just like I was but unlike the rest of the crowd.[10] Though people may suggest that children are dualists, they also appear – perhaps more strongly – to be immersed, completely at times, in their bodies and in their activities. One of the joys of child-hood, from the outside at least, is exactly the way in which young kids are lost in action, whether in play, or in the joy of skipping or kicking a ball.

With Möbius Celia felt cut off from immersion in action in the body and so cut off from much of what it is to be a child. After all, as she said, children have a different language from adults, a body and facial language, revealed during play rather than during speech. She was faced with a dawning realization of her difference and of the gap between herself, and her collection of body parts, and her peers. The polite grown-up conversations with adults, 'Adults were my friends, not children,' the books and her internal dialogues may have been of little consolation.

Chapter 5

Part of me

The experiences of Charlie and Gemma are largely absent from their stories, as one might expect from ones so young. Celia, in contrast and looking back as an adult, remembers how Möbius had complex effects as she grew up, as school and social life outside the family became more important. The next four chapters contain the narratives of grown-ups who have lived with their Möbius for 30 to 50 years or so. Some were young, when awareness of impairment was less widespread in society and support and assistance less available, and this may explain, at least in part, the starkness of some of their accounts. The first person, Lizzie, is in her early thirties. I had arranged to meet her in a Dublin hotel lobby. When I arrived I saw the top of a head buried in a book; as she scanned each line, her head moved back and forth. I knew her by her reading style; without movement of the eyes in the head some "Möbians" become dizzy reading.

We went out for coffee, walking through the busy city streets. She was nervous, never having talked about her life before; she walked without talking, a little apart from me, so I kept my distance too. After coffee and some small talk we went back to the hotel lobby. It was noisy – a Dublin hen night was refuelling nearby – and I had to strain to hear her soft voice. After College, she told me, where she read philosophy, she did a course in office management. She had worked for AHEAD, the Association for Higher Education Access and Disability and is now with Dublin City Council Corporate Services in the Communication Section, in a big office overlooking the River Liffey. She edits a children's newsletter called *Classmate*.

A solitary twin

'When I was 4, I looked in a mirror and looked at Sarah and I knew something was different and I asked my Dad and he said, "Arrhh, don't worry about it." I never looked across at Sarah and wondered why I was not like her. You just grow up to accept it as it is. I have never said to Sarah, "Why am I not like you?"

'I stammered and I could not say the word "twin". It was easier for me to say she was my sister than my twin. We were not in the same class and I consider her more a sister than a twin. We don't even look alike; Sarah is tall with curly hair, so we are very different – you would not know we are sisters, let alone twins.

'I was very happy with my family and friends. My childhood was fine. I was a good girl. I had a twin sister to stand up for me even though she was in a different class. My mother wanted us in the same class but they said, keep Lizzie back a year. At the time Mum was upset but, looking back, I had my own friends and I was not always tagging along with my sister. She would come home from school and tell what had happened in my class. She was very outgoing as a child. Sarah would talk to everyone, she was so extrovert. I was much quieter.

'At that time I did not know I had a disability.[1] I was never bullied. Others with Möbius have said they were, but I was not. Perhaps it was the school. There were some children who my parents said would not play with me, but I never noticed because I had my friends too.'

Lizzie's family did not know she had Möbius until she was 12. They never made much of her problem anyway. 'They didn't stop me from having a life.' She could not ride a bike because of her poor balance. Even then her parents never said she could not have one, though, in the end, she had a scooter instead.

Lizzie still has problems with balance and turning.

'I can go from right to left OK, but if I go left to right I have problems. It is partly because I have to turn my head. As a kid I would bump into things. Even now I cannot see down as I walk because of the eyes. I go to body balance in the gym and this is helping, but it is all down the left side, like my face [her Möbius is unilateral, on the left, and her left hand lacks a finger or two]. I am alright going up an escalator but feel I am falling off on the way down. However, I have mastered it. When I was a child we used to go to Wicklow and scramble over rocks and I always had problems.'

Lizzie has not begun to drive yet for the same reason. Without movement of the eyes in the head it is difficult not only to see around widely enough but also to judge speed and distance. But she is beginning to take this on, driving with her father on a beach to start with. Many of the parts of driving, changing gear, starting, stopping, and hill starts are less of a problem than the judgements of speed.

Just a word

The teens were difficult; Lizzie became aware of being different, and found that she had to work twice as hard as the others to keep up.

'That time was tricky. I gave my Mum a hard time, in part because I became aware of my disability. I was not like my peers with facial expressions. I have close friends now, very close, but back then I would just read books. I always have books, I retreated into them. I would go upstairs and read. At 13, I was reading *Persuasion*.

'Möbius was a label put on me at 12, when I saw my ophthalmic surgeon. I had had an operation on my eye at 11. The doctors knew about Möbius when I was a couple of days old but they did not tell my parents. They would have liked to have known so they could explain to people what I had. Dad did research on it in the library but Möbius wasn't in the medical books. In Ireland only 10 to 15 people have it. There are three down in Cork and a teenager in Dublin plus me; that's five people I know. I often watch people's faces to see if they are like me. Faces are life, they talk, and they might have a burn or something wrong, or a cancer, when you see it you see their life. Then I got on with my life, Möbius was just a word. I accepted me for what I was.

'At 17, my parents took me to a doctor about my hand. But there was no point. He said he could do an operation on my face, but I would have to grind my teeth to make a smile. I realized how different I was and I thought I had coped that long and thought, "no operation."

'I loved going to school, but 13 is a hard age; I was neither child nor adult. To have the Möbius added one thing more. I hated my teenage years and was very quiet and would not go back there. I always wanted to go to school but I was very quiet, though I played hockey and went to drama for a year. I was not into fashion and make-up or clothes. I would go into town and buy a book. All teenagers are different.

'My sister was going out and was extrovert. I learnt the hard way that the more people you know, the more you have to go out with. My best friend went to America for a year and then I saw less of my friends. However, I had two or three very close friends. Now I have different sets of friends and see them regularly. I don't go out with the same group and don't rely on one friend to go out with. In my teens I did, and now realize that it is better to have lots of friends so that I am not relying on the same person.'

Repeating

Throughout Lizzie's teenage years she found schoolwork difficult and she had to repeat several years. Each time, she was left behind by her year group of friends, just as she had been left behind by her twin sister.

'At college, there would be coffee breaks and there was no choice but to talk to someone beside you. The first two months I was a bit wary, out of my comfort zone. Then, when I repeated a year, I had no friends. I went to a different school and could not make that connection and no one knew I had no friends at the college. I knew no one. How could I make friends? I found that very hard.

'I did not even tell my parents or sister. I only told her a couple of years ago. She said, "What of your friends from the Institute?" and I said I had none. I was 19. I was doubting myself. I spent a year not talking to anyone, especially over the first two months. I asked someone there and they said, "You've got to talk to me." It was new people and in the end there was a girl from my school and I knew her, though she was a year above because I repeated a year. Towards the end of the year I did make some friends. It was self-esteem.

'I was very determined. I repeated in school and then in College I repeated each year. I found it hard; I always had to work so hard. It is not ability. I knew I could do it. But even in school, though I did not struggle, I panicked the first time I did my leaving certificate.'

Hard to meet

Last year, Lizzie went to a Möbius Support Group meeting for the first time. She found the support group daunting. 'I walked into a room full of people who looked like me.' It made her realize how very strange it had been to not grow up with people who looked like her. Previously, she had only met a little girl of 11 who had had smile surgery.

'She was not forthcoming and I was 15 years older and how could I ask a child what it was like and she could not know what I was going through? I did not know what she was going through as a child since as a child I did not grow up with a disability. I was a normal kid going to school and doing drama. I swam. I did not sit and say I am different; what would people have thought of me?

'I did not know what I wanted from the meeting. I wanted a person the same age as me. I shied away from the first few hours and then someone said, "You have to go over and meet someone." So a person introduced me to a woman seven years younger than me and we just talked in general and then I began to open up. Nicki and I are friends now and are in contact regularly by email and text. I went over to visit her in April and saw her in August.

'In a room [full of people] looking like me, having only seen one in my life, this was not real. Nicki, my new friend, understood. To go into a room like that as a person who looks like everybody else was scary, especially when I wasn't used to it. Just because we have Möbius does not mean we will become friends. We talked about our reactions to other people and how they react to us. We compared experiences, for instance, what you do when someone says, "Smile," the reactions of other people, doing up shoelaces, etc.

'I don't know how I feel. Last week was an eye-opener. I went over to see Nicki and we went to the pub on a Saturday and I met Tory on the Sunday. Those two knew each other and when Tory opened the door they hugged each other and I stepped back and became very quiet. I had never actually been out like that. We all look the same but I would never go out with another. In the shopping centre, watching people look at us and on the bus, I never had had that before. I felt claustrophobic and by Monday I needed my own space. I am never with people who look like me and go out with friends and go to the pub or cinema, or the gym, or work. I had never experienced that. For 26 years of my life I knew no one with it. I always believed that the support group would be good. I would still go and want them in my life but I don't need them every week or every month.

'When I was there we socialized, all Möbius together. But I have other friends and it was kind of weird. I want my own identity – and have it – and Möbius is but one part of my life. I am pleased to live in Ireland and to have space here from the group. It was hard to meet so many people that were of a similar way. I get tired and if I don't eat or have cups of coffee I get tired.

'Some of the phone calls Nicki had were from people with Möbius. If I had had that, as a child, I would have been different. I could have talked with them. I never had it and I just got on with it; my parents and teachers got on with it and so did my friends. I was not singled out. Nicki and her friends all gravitate towards each other and have shared experiences. I never had that and did not know how to relate to them at that stage. I wished I had a support group because they have more confidence.'

At the conference there had been a physical therapist who specializes in Bell's palsy and she arranged a meeting in Manchester for those with Möbius. Lizzie went and stayed with Nicki. There she decided to try facial stimulation, to see if building up the muscles on her weak side might reduce the asymmetry and, even better, give her more controlled movement.[2]

'The facial stimulation gives me a shock every couple of seconds ... I've bought it now, though the last months I have been so busy I have not used it. I have had movement of my right side for a long time and maybe it now moves a little on the left. I sit at home on the PC at home and have it on at the same time.'

It is too early to know if it will be useful.

Returned to Möbius

Most of the time Lizzie does not live with Möbius, but occasionally others, unthinkingly and unfeelingly, return her to it. She mentioned several episodes she finds difficult to put behind her.

'My friends were grand and never mentioned anything. I felt more different than they felt [I was]. At one dance I asked a boy to dance with me and he said he would not because of my left hand and that was the first time I knew I was different. I was terrified.

'Once, my cousin, when aged 3, turned around and said I talk funny and have a different face. My sister was there and said don't worry about it. He is 21 now and is grand. I felt his parents could have explained. That experience awakened me into realizing that I had a disability. As a child, I have no memory of being different.

'When I was 13 [I met] a guy aged 15 who had been burnt; I thought that people would have to look beyond the surface to get to know him, for looks aren't everything. If I see a person with an abnormality, I get to know them as people. I believe that we all have a hidden disability and we just get to know people within the inside.

'A couple of months ago I started doing voluntary work for the Special Olympics and I went into the room and said, "Hello!" and one of the volunteers asked if I had come for the Basketball and I said, "No, I am a volunteer." She was only 17 and you have to understand that teenagers may not be tactful. But I was recently in Paris and I was sitting on the plane over in the emergency seat and the air hostess asked me to move and did not give me an explanation, so I got up and went to another seat.

'But then I asked another hostess and said that I had walked onto the plane and this has not happened before and I needed no assistance. But they said I was not able-bodied enough. I thought they were insensitive. I reckon she saw my face and my hand and made a judgement.'

Years ago that would have been the end of it, with Lizzie living with her sadness and frustration. Now, as an adult, she took them on.

'I got onto their website and complained. I clicked onto "reduced mobility" where they go on about wheelchair access. I can understand that, but is this how they define reduced mobility? I did not fit into any of their categories and yet they would not allow me to sit there. I wrote to them and they said they had high standards and it would not happen again. They would not ask my sister to move. They assumed because my face was not right I was not right.'

Recently there was an incident at her gym.

'I was in a step class and I could not keep up and the teacher asked who thought it was too fast and only I put up my hand. She did not acknowledge me and continued with the class. I get frustrated at times, not to be able to do things as quickly as other people. Trying to explain to the instructor that I just want to do step class without struggling was difficult.'

Banging doors

These things, though infrequent, bring her back to Möbius with a start and mean that she has learnt that she can never completely be free. 'Just once I would like to be able to be like everybody else.' But things are getting better.

'I am growing more confident and in the last few years I have considered who I am. Most of the time, it is fine. I live a life, I work, I go to the gym, and travel and read. I would never buy a best-seller. I have read all Austen and all the classics from Dickens to Marquez and I am in a book club at work. But I have not got past the first paragraph of Ulysses, which is a shame, being a Dubliner.

'I do not avoid faces. If I am in the pub at night, I have to look at everyone and I take a moment to recognize them. It looks like I am staring but it is not. I cannot move my eyes so I have to look. People and faces are interesting. At times I worry that by looking at them they will look at me. Faces are more fascinating to me; there is a story behind every face. I hate using "normal". If you had a burn on your face, or were tall and skinny, the world makes judgments. I try not to make judgments.

'I don't go, "Wow, I am a twin." My sister cannot pick up things about me more than others. All my family know when I am angry or upset; I bang doors. I find it hard when I cannot smile and seeing other people reacting to that. I have started salsa dancing classes and people react to my left hand with a sympathetic face but now in the class they don't seem to notice.'

She is still frustrated when she cannot get her point across.

'I cannot smile, but would like to be able to smile like everyone else. I cannot show I am smiling: I give a blank look; it could be anything, smiling, angry. But people still know when I am happy. I laugh with my friends and when I am upset I cry and I get angry at home and with friends. I express in different ways. I slam doors but I go quiet too, when upset. My friends know when I feel various moods. When being photographed it is better for me to keep a straight face since when I smile the [right] side goes up so it is better to keep still, even though my friends love it. I know my face does not express. I am concerned sometimes that I may be misunderstood, so I do tell them. The smile was a bigger issue, when younger and a teenager.

'In the last few years I have begun to think about life. In the past it sort of passed me by and I did not know too much about it. I was sometimes distant towards people and I wanted to know if it was part of Möbius or just other people's reactions. There are a lot of things which Möbius people can do, but only by adapting. For years I wanted shoe laces but could not tie them. Now in the gym I just use Velcro. Before, every five minutes I would have to retie them. I cannot move my eyes and have to use my head; I read by moving my head.'

I mentioned that I had recognized her this way as she read in the lobby. She laughed.

'At the support group I needed to see whether others had the same problems and what was me and what was due to Möbius. Everyone has different symptoms and I needed to find out about myself. At the support group I just wanted to know if most people had the same patterns of thought and feeling and why.'

Becoming

She returned to the air hostess and the girl at the Olympic event. Small things, perhaps, in the grand scheme of things, things which might be laughed off, if only she had the resilience and confidence, but things which still, several years later, were affecting her.

'When the 17-year-old said that to me, I forced back tears. There were other people around who knew I was a volunteer and yet they did not say anything. Things can be grand for a couple of months and then bang, something happens and someone says something and you want to say, "I am not like that." I may have reduced mobility but I am physically strong, robust, and healthy. Able-bodied is being able to walk with two feet in front of you. I walked onto that plane and it was so insensitive.'[3]

More than a personal affront, it was the sheer unfairness which hurt.

'As a child I didn't know I had Möbius, I was just me. It got bad in adolescence. I was quiet and hid away. Whether I was quiet because of the Möbius or not, I don't know. I did not like being a teenager. In my mid twenties I began to become me, and say, "I am me and I don't care what anybody else thinks of me," and I got on with my life. I have coped this far.

'I learnt an awful lot in my first conference. I needed more interaction with other adults, just to see what they were going through and to understand from those with similar experience. It is a part of my life, and it is not going to take over. As a child it was not much of a part but then at 12 it was, when I was told I had Möbius. I still got on with it and was tough. I had a bad stammer as a child and was self-conscious of it. In my twenties I have coped this far, and now I am older I have to find out

about me. It is now less of a part than it was. I don't have to phone the conference people every week with the same condition … That is not me.'

I mentioned one person who was nearly undone by the support
group. Her Möbius was such a small part of her and yet, at the support
group, it was all about Möbius.

'It is a small part of me and I don't want to be just that.[4] I have lived a life,
31 years, not only being my face. Why should I suddenly be submerged into
a situation all about Möbius? There are other things. The worst of Möbius is
that people see you and think there is something wrong with you. All my
friends know and lots of people are grand. I don't think there is anything
bad about it … It is me. The people who stare or react in a negative way are
people that you don't want to know anyway.'

Her face was, however, different and this visible difference precludes
her fading into the background and becoming inconspicuous, except
with her good friends and family.

'A lot of people remember me that I don't remember at all. People come up
to me and say, "Hi, Lizzie!" and I don't remember them. A schoolfriend
came up to me when I was having lunch and she saw me and said, "Hi!"
After 11 years, lots of people recognize me because I have an unusual face.
Then I sometimes mistake people. In college I said, "Hello!" to someone
and it was the wrong person.[5] The worst of Möbius is that people see you
and think there is something wrong with you.'

One might wish to be remembered for many things, but for having
facial immobility is probably not high on the list, especially when trying
to emerge from Möbius and define one's identity independent of it.
Lizzie was getting there.

'I am part of a gang who don't have Möbius and it is good that way. In
the last two years I am more assertive. The gym problem I mentioned –
years ago I would not have said anything. In fact, I was shocked by what
I said. That is not normally me and I did apologize for what I said.

'My problem has been being quiet. Can you change a quiet person?
I am starting to be more assertive over the last 10 years. I live at home …
Now, I am saving to get a house or flat with my sister. I find now it is claustrophobic and my mum keeps coming into my room. We hope to move
out soon. I will live with my twin sister. That's the next thing. We will probably kill each other – everyone needs space. I do need to get away.

'We are all different. I could not care less what other people look like.
Because I have an impairment, I do not judge people by appearance
as much as others. I couldn't change my face and could not change my

fingers, so I went on and did whatever others do too. I am stronger for it. I have to work harder but I will not give up. Everyone knows me as Lizzie. People who want to be my friends are my friends. That's it.'

With that we finished. I walked her to the end of the street where, surrounded once more by all the noise and life of Dublin, we parted. I wanted to hug her and tell her how much more of a life was waiting. Instead we just shook hands.

~~

In the next chapter we meet James, a man now in his sixties, whose Möbius has been a constant influence, despite its presence being hidden from him for many years.

Chapter 6

The spectator[1]

James began at his beginning.

'I was born in 1939, the third of six brothers and sisters. They had to find a way of feeding me. Eventually they used the inside of a fountain pen and dripped it into my mouth. Each feed took two hours, and if I was sick they did it again. My mother had a nurse who lived in at each of her confinements. For mine, she stayed far longer than usual. I was also tongue-tied, so the family doctor, who was a surgeon, did a series of operations releasing it.'

He does not remember any awareness of being different until, when 8, he went to the village school. He was very late going because of Möbius.

'Occasionally, at home, I used to salivate when I talked and sometimes I was accused of spitting when there was no intention to do so. [At school] they used to say that I had spat in the cocoa or that I was spitting at some other boy and I'd get into trouble. I don't think it had occurred to me inside the family environment that there was anything particularly unusual about me. What made me realize I was different was the questioning about my funny face.

'At the age of 11, when I went to the grammar school, I used to be asked why do I cry when I eat. I still do and have to wipe my face. I was teased, partly because my father was on the staff and partly because my older brother was a senior pupil. It may not have had anything to do with me and I think I misunderstood that. I was an object of curiosity and interest, not simply because of what I was but because of who I was.

'I did, however, begin to become aware of difficulties in communicating with people. For instance in those early years at grammar school, some people didn't understand me. If I put my hand up in class because I knew the answer the teacher wouldn't ask me. I felt neglected.

'I had speech therapy for two or three years. She helped me considerably in slowing down and separating the words. She taught me to put the final consonant onto the end of a word to help people understand what I was saying. By the end of my time at grammar school, masters would say that whilst it wasn't exactly a pleasure to talk to me at least they could understand what I was saying.

'It was a single-sex school and we lived about seven miles outside town. Whatever difficulties I had because of my face, I also had the difficulty in socializing because my friends lived in town and there was only one bus home and I had to be on it. It was only when I was in the sixth form that I started going to one or two out-of-hours gatherings and I started to get about. I was afraid and in awe of girls for a long time.

'I was fairly placid as a child but I sometimes remember my face working for me rather than against me. If I did something wrong, I'd say, "It wasn't me, Mummy, it was him." My brother was 13 months younger and I would be believed. I soon learned that my facial problem allowed me deception. I've never played poker. As a child I did a lot of reading, which suggests a certain solitary quality. In my teens I read Hardy, perhaps not the ideal thing at that stage either for me or for others around me. I would be by myself in the book, burying my face in it.

'I had always had it in mind to offer myself for ordination and when I was around 18 I had an interview and was offered a place at Cambridge as long as I was accepted by the Church as a candidate for ordination. So I went to a Church of England Selection Conference, which recommended in turn that I should be taken on. Then I had the medical in Chester; I failed on the grounds of speech. The standing and walking was also thought to be too much of an obstacle. It was a great shock to have passed the interview and yet have the doctor turn me down. I remember that. But there was a second opinion built into the process and I went to see a Harley Street man at the Church's expense. He said, "Well, Mr Brown, I can understand you, and you walked across my extensive consulting room well enough." So he reversed the decision.

I asked him how he viewed his face and himself in those days. He answered tangentially.

'I have a notion, which has stayed with me over much of my life – that it is possible to live in your head; entirely in my head. Whether that came out of my facial problem, I don't know. I was very introspective. I divided people into two categories: those who didn't want to have anything to do with me for various reasons and those who did.

'I think I had a low idea of self-worth. Thinking about it and reflecting upon it, I think in a sense a Christian shouldn't think too highly of himself in any case, though I realize you do not have to belittle yourself either. I haven't related these things to my face particularly and that's why I haven't been speaking about it. I just haven't focused anything on the face. I had feelings of low self-esteem and loneliness and isolation in company, where I wasn't with anyone particularly, and I had the feeling, say, at a long table during a meal, say in my Cambridge College, that the conversation divided around me and I was left on my own to eat my food and I was happy to do that – but not really happy. These feelings I have lived with, in my head. I always found it difficult to break in.

'It is only very recently that the whole area of non-verbal communication has even come to my attention. I know now that since I put out a reduced range of signals, I receive back a similarly reduced range. Is he going to know me today, is he going to speak to me today, as I approach someone? As I go about in the street I see people coming towards me and I can tell if they're going to get ready to speak to me if I speak to them, but it's taken me a long time to latch onto that fact.

'I think I was lonely at Cambridge. Again I don't relate it to my face, although it may be pertinent. I lived in digs in my first year; I made one or two friends amongst the theological students. I didn't join a lot of societies. The first year I was quite lonely. The second and third years I was resident in college and that was far better – I was in the centre of things.'

James seemed not to relate these difficulties to his face at all, but to a deeper, far deeper, level; to him and his inadequacies. I asked to what extent he thought his lack of facial expression affected this.

'I don't really think in those terms even now. You just accept that that's the way you are without asking why.

'People tend to take everything I say seriously. [Because] I can't smile, I can't always communicate a joke – it's all to do with facial expression and I've got into trouble because of that. I say things with a straight face. Once a young woman asked me what I'd do as a curate if a young baby cried at a baptism and I said, "Oh, I'd hit its head on the side of the font," and she went to the Vicar with great anger and upset because she didn't realize that I was joking.'

'Some days I could go out and see four or five people; some days I'd sit at home, not able to do it. I interpreted that as being not very good at the job. I was judgmental on myself about this.'

Becoming a priest was partially his calling and partly to please his mother. But he also accepts that he was looking for a fixed social role to play in front of others. He enjoyed ministering to older people especially, say, in their homes and taking funerals. It was more difficult, for example, chairing meetings. This was not only because he was more exposed, but because it was difficult for him to impose his own view to get his way. Going out to meet new people, perhaps a new family moving into the parish, required a great, conscious effort.

'I had a social role, which to some extent I hid behind: well, I thought I did, though it is in that area that I became uncertain. I lost that sense of myself. Perhaps I lost it so long ago but I became aware of the fact that I didn't have that sense of myself.'

Before elaborating he moved on, to his wife.

'I met Anne in my first parish. She was one of the congregation and I came to know her because I was lodging with someone who was a friend. Anne used to call on my landlady and was thrust at me. I found the first few days after we met very difficult, but I had a very practical reason for persisting: the landlady had left for six weeks and I found it difficult to cope. Of course I was taken with her as well and have always been very glad that we both persisted. Once we began to relax together, then we both were fairly equally committed and there was a reciprocity, which was entirely different.

'I think initially I was thinking I was in love with her. It was some time later when I realized that I really felt in love.'

'At Cambridge, and later, I think I survived by being withdrawn or introspective. I made a virtue of keeping myself to myself. I think I rather liked not being like the others. You can become very perverse. For far too long that's what I did. I liked being not like the others. I gained some solace from it.'

He accepts that there was an element of self-deception in this. 'I got into various difficulties later on because it wasn't a way of coping over a lifetime. It worked for quite a long time. Maybe it worked until my mother died, in 1980 when I was in my forties.' Then he began to reflect on that relationship and what he really wanted to do. He realized how unhappy he was working as a parish priest and for a while he was depressed. He saw a psychiatrist who was also a priest. More recently, for the first time, he has been talking with a spiritual director who asked him about anger, and whether he might be angry with God. For the first time he thought that, 'Yes, I have been angry.' But still he did not relate its origin to the face.

'Part of the problem is that you're not supposed to express anger. If you're angry you're told to stop it; but it is a powerful emotion and I realize that now and I think it has done a lot of damage in the past for instance in my attitude to work and parishioners.'

After the death of his mother he came to think that he had to choose between the role of being a vicar and being – or finding – himself.

'Had I ever been myself? I was losing me as a priest but trying desperately to recover just me, James. This is a new thought. Perhaps I had spent my life as someone else in order not to be me. Me is something I see in the mirror. I have always had a difficulty with mirrors and photographs. I don't like being confronted by me.

'Even though I realize that what I see is not me, even in a mirror it's an image, a partial image. I don't want to look in a mirror, and apart from shaving I never do. I avoid them, and photographs. As a curate or a vicar, folk say, "Well, let's have a photograph," after a baptism or a wedding, and you do it. And you say, "Well, that's not me, that's the Vicar." I have spent a lot of my life hiding behind a dog collar. Any development that has taken place more recently came about in part through the Möbius support group and seeing that there are other folk and other families that have it much worse and have had to struggle much harder than me.

'It is easier now to talk about myself; I had never previously talked to anyone very much. I love the Church of England and there are fine men amongst its leaders but they don't really want to know. They may ask you how you are and its OK if you say, "Very well," but if you say, "I'm about to drop this tea tray," they don't know what to do. Or they give you the impression that they'd say, "Well drop it and then we can do something. But before then we're powerless."

'I did go through a period in the late 1980s when I was quite desperate and I would describe it in terms of, "I am going to drop this tea tray." Perhaps to get attention but I didn't really want to drop it, I just wanted someone to listen and do something. Those problems I didn't explicitly relate to the problems of the Möbius syndrome. But they do relate to the more general need to find myself, which in turn relates to the Möbius. Perhaps I did turn my back on self-expression. Perhaps self-expression was beyond me. It was just quite enough to get by day to day.'

It was only quite late in his life, in his fifties, that he realized that he had Möbius syndrome and that he was not alone. His mother-in-law saw an article in a paper about it and sent him the cutting. When he read the story, about a little boy who can't smile, it was the first time he realized that there were others.

'Meeting the Möbius Group has had a good, very positive effect on me. I was 53 and I had never even heard the name Möbius. It had never really occurred to me, nor had I wondered consciously, how many like me are there out there. I hadn't thought of it but I certainly may have turned my back on my face, much more than I had ever realized or supposed. This idea I mentioned earlier of attempting to live behind it, may well be an escape from something I found intolerable.'

In talking about dropping the tea tray, James had used an example of a sudden loud explosion of frustration or anger. This raised the question of his emotional experience, whether a certain transient happiness, or fear, say, was possible without their bodily expression.

'I think there's a lot of dissociation. But I think I get trapped in my mind or my head. I sort of think happy or I think sad, not really saying or recognizing actually feeling happy or feeling sad. Perhaps I have had a difficulty in recognizing that which I'm putting a name to is not a thought at all but it is a feeling; maybe I have to intellectualize mood. I have to say, "This thought is a happy thought and, therefore, I am happy."

'I think also that I have a fear of being out of control with emotions, feeling something that I can't manage. I have also found it very difficult to communicate feelings throughout my life, whether as a child or with my wife, though I think I am getting better at it now. I don't really know how I communicate happiness or sadness. That's a very hard question. Some people cry when they're sad. I don't. I sometimes felt that I would like to be able to cry but you see I am not really able to cry, my tears can come but there's nothing else. My tears only flow when I eat. I am afraid of such feelings. I try and shut them off.'

In his ministry he has seen many things which are sad and has told the person that he felt very sorry for them, when he was thinking that rather than feeling it.

'Of course, since I have never been able to move the face, I've never associated movement of the face with feeling of an emotion. If I have expressed any emotion I must have spoken it or I might put my arm around someone.'

In his job, he was not required to feel what he was trying to express. 'I've often thought of myself as a spectator rather than as a participant.' As a vicar, he was a professional spectator and maybe it was by leaving the parochial ministry that he was exploring his non-spectator self with and beyond Möbius. He agreed, to a point.

'Yes, but people; they are their faces. I think I would like to be my face. I am beginning to want to be my face. I may become more assertive without being more aggressive. In the past, I have often had an idea but not managed to do something, whereas now I am beginning to do something, whether it's the idea to ring someone up or send them a card, I actually follow it through. I am becoming more pro-active. I am entering into the world more than in the past.

'I can read faces but I can't give a face in return. In that sense, I am invisible or blank. I may have traded on the blankness from time to time. I have sometimes thought, when I have felt low, if only other people knew what I am thinking. Other people may not want to have thoughts that they're feeling portrayed to others. I know that none of my thoughts will ever be seen by others on my face.'

James showed me a passage from the Bible which had sustained him, said to relate to Christ's coming, Isaiah 53, beginning at verse 2:

He had no beauty, no majesty to draw our eyes,
No grace to make us delight in Him;
His form, disfigured, lost all the likeness of a man, his beauty changed
    beyond human semblance.
He was despised, he shrank from the sight of men, tormented and
    humbled by suffering;
We despised him. We held him of no account, the thing from which
    men turn away their eyes.
He was afflicted, and did not open his mouth … He was cut off from
    the world of living men.

'It's only in recent times that I've dared to think of that passage in terms of myself. I could not obviously claim all of that but I do feel that I fit in somewhere. Several years ago I would never have thought of seeing myself there and if I had done so I'd have thought, "That's wrong, that's blasphemous." But now I think I understand those words better and they have a personal involvement for me and they have a message, which is: "This is how I am and I must accept it, can accept it," and in being related to me they are very positive words too.

'In the past I wouldn't have put my face or my experiences with this. I see that now, much more clearly. Thirty years ago I didn't, it was inappropriate; I was denying the face, my face. I think I am beginning to feel that I can think that way, realize my face and almost in some way be glad of it or accept it.

'I now realize that some things which may have been due to the condition I felt were just down to me. Rather than saying that the condition has made life difficult, I have been saying I have made life difficult. It was my fault. I have failed.

'One of the things I think that's happening now is that I have a sense of becoming freer; freer in the sense of becoming more myself, not playing a role. I certainly wanted to try and explore me behind the mask of the priesthood. If you say where does "me" now reside, I think I am slowly coming out of my head. I am not sure I can locate where I am but I don't think I am entirely in my head or even my mind. I have an expression of living "a life of the mind", but I do accept that the mind is not easily able to communicate its thoughts or even its feelings. I think I was out of touch with my feelings, or I suppressed a lot of them.

'I have been told I am a very placid person. My sister said, "You never cried, you were a very good child in that sense." I had all these things, operations, manipulations, splints but I can't know now how much was a placidness of nature and how much was a suppression of feeling.

'The lack of the smile is a scourge in the teenage years and is more of a problem than anything else, more than the eating in public; being misunderstood, not being able to register recognition or salutation and particularly with girls.'

As he said, it is only recently that he has become aware of non-verbal communication, only recently that he has used his arms in gesture; before he would keep them by his side, tools for working, not parts for expressing and sharing. Only recently has he considered his sense of self and where it resides. For much of his life it has been in his head, and only now has it begun to inhabit his body. Now he is exploring how the further he is in his body, the closer he is to the world and to others. He used to be accused of staring at people because he has to turn his head towards them to see them, so he stopped looking. More recently one of his brothers said that he was looking at him more. Now, in his fifties and sixties, his journey outwards to the world is under way.

Chapter 7

Elastic between us

Möbius syndrome is manifest in face and eye problems and by hand and foot maldevelopments. In addition, it will be remembered, there is also evidence of more cognitive problems; learning difficulties and autism, though the prevalence of these is uncertain. I went to see Alison and Peggy.

Three sisters

Alison is coming up to 50; her mother, Peggy, spoke first.

> 'She was born in this house and could not open her eyes or feed. The doctor did not know what to do; they took her off to hospital the next day. I was in bed for two weeks, as you were then, and could do nothing. After 10 days she came home with no advice. No one said anything.'

Alison could not suck, so Will, Peggy's husband, found a bottle to feed her. Breastfeeding was usual then, so it was fortunate that a woman opposite was using bottle-feed milk, and they borrowed some of this. He made a large hole in the teat and poured it down. Alison occasionally choked, but at least she was feeding. After a few days, the midwife stopped coming.

At 18 months, she went to the Eye Hospital to have her eyelids stitched back: the skin was so loose it threatened to obstruct her vision.[1] In hospital she was distraught when they left, desperately shouting her only words, 'Mummy! Daddy!' When she came home two weeks later she did not speak for a month. She was generally slow to pick up words, though once she really started talking, at 4 or so, she never shut up. Her parents had no problem understanding her, despite her Möbius.[2] Peggy continued,

> 'The worst part was taking Alison out. A cousin had seen a baby with eyes all over the place with mental subnormality and Alison's were the same. I would take her shopping and people would say, "How awful."'

Nursery school was fine but by the time she was 5, and ready for proper school, she was so hyperactive that mainstream schools would not take her. Instead she had one-to-one teaching at home and then went to a number of special schools. When even they found her too difficult, her mother, at the end of her wits, wrote to her MP. He arranged a school for Alison. She was still hyperactive though and, in the end, aged 7 or so, a doctor gave her tryptizol, a tranquillizer, to calm her down.

At this school, she boarded during the week and came home for weekends. One Sunday, having dropped her back at school, Will and Peggy forgot something and went back. They found Alison locked in her room. They immediately took her home.

> 'We knew nothing and to us, she was just Alison. Others thought she was mentally handicapped. We treated her like the others and she joined in with our other two girls. But Alison needed so much attention that the others brought themselves up. She was into everything as the others got on with their schoolwork.'

At the next special school she stayed several years and her mother and father thought she was getting on very well. Then, at one Open Day, the head said she was the worst girl they had ever had. Her mother felt attacked. After that she went to an adult training centre, where she stayed for the next 25 years.

She did every course they ran, from art and design and embroidery, to carpentry, picture framing, and leather work. Some were to a high level, with Alison receiving City and Guilds Certificates. Recently she was given a Life-Long Learning Award and a cheque for £50 in recognition of this.[3] The college was brilliant because it mainstreamed those with learning difficulties, but once she had done every course she was asked to leave. Now, a succession of various centres occupy her time but she does not learn; at one she was filling envelopes and at another putting screws into things. She did not like that: 'I got bored. I am too able for that.'

She also works in an Old People's Home and for that was awarded a New Year's Honour from the local Centre for Voluntary Work. At one centre, a teacher was keen on athletics and, as a result, Alison has been to several Special Olympics.

'I've got lots of medals, in running, darts, javelin, and swimming, and I went to France and the Isle of Wight. In the 800m, there were two of us and I did my socks up and still came first.'

Alison continued, 'I get the fruit out; take the cups to the kitchen.' This was at the Old People's Home. She still goes there on a Thursday. 'I did a course in hairdressing.'

There had been the sniff of romance once. Alison volunteered: 'Paul was in respite. He wanted assistance with a toilet during the night … 'He made Alison an offer,' her mother said, '… he could not see very well.' 'Just as well.' Alison shot back. Whatever else, her sense of humour was working. She showed me her book, beautifully written out in long hand.

Alison's Memories

(Reproduced with permission)

Chapter 1

When I was 18 months old I went to the Eye Hospital for an operation on my eyes and eyelids.

When I was 4 years old I went to Nursery School. One of the nursery nurses was Mrs Spicer who looked after me. When I was 5 I had to leave. But I could not go to school because I was hyperactive so Mrs Spicer offered to come to my house for one hour each day and she taught me how to read. When I was 7 I went to a Junior Training Centre …

I went to the next Boarding School in September. I was there for about 6 weeks. At half term I was sent home and as there was no return date given Mom phoned the school and was told that they didn't want me back as they could not cope with me. Mom and Dad were frantic as I had so many changes so they went to see our local MP. He wrote to say there was a place was a Special School and I went there until I was 16. Then I transferred to a Training Centre where I still go.

Chapter 2 The School

I went into Mrs Lee's class. She was very tough and shouted a lot. I made friends with Joyce Smith (she had an artificial arm) and Beth White.

My other teachers were Mr Best, Mr Gibbs, Mr Hansen, Kathy Reeves, John Craven and Mrs Sparrow. Her nickname was Sparrow legs. Miss Shreve was the headmistress.

I did PE, I liked that with Mrs West.
I also did cooking with Mrs Salt. I made cakes.
I also did pottery with Mr Boyce. I made a dish.
And I did woodwork and metalwork and some sewing. I made a make-up bag.

One of my teachers got married and she became my friend. She used to come to my house with Mr Best. When I left the school they left the area and I lost contact.

Chapter 3 My holidays

Mom and Dad took me on holidays with my two sisters. We used to have a caravan or a flat at the seaside. We went to Weston-super-Mare and went in an aeroplane. We went to Crimdon Dene in County Durham where my Gran lived.

I also went to Rhos on Sea. A lady from social services took me there for a week while Mom and Dad had a break to see my Gran. And we had holidays at Butlins Holiday Camp.

At about 12 years old my Mom and Dad took me to a place in Wales. It was a lovely place and I had 2 weeks there while my Mom and Dad had a different holiday. I went there every year and made friends with Pugsley and Fred who looked after me. [It was a Mencap Holiday Home.] I still write to Pugsley and visited her last year. She and Fred are now married with two young boys. The Hall closed in the 1980s so I couldn't go any more. Now I go to the Hostel while Mom and Dad go somewhere. I used to go to Daisy Bank. That was nice. I was happy there, but the short-term care stopped. This year I am going on an adventure holiday in France.

Chapter 4

When I started at the next school Mrs Moses was the manager. I was with Mrs Wright and Mrs George. They were very kind and I was kept busy doing handicraft.

I have been there now for 19 years and I have seen a lot of changes. I started off making coat hangers with Mrs Wright. She died and I was with Mrs George. We made cushions and snakes. We used to have trips, which was nice.

Mr Goater left to go to another centre and Mr Glover came, he was interested in the special Olympics.

I had a very special friend, he was a supervisor called Freddie Vaughan. He was very kind and helpful to me. He had diabetes and one day he was taken very ill and was in hospital. I used to visit him and he died. I was very sad.

Things began to change. Mrs George retired and all the staff seemed to be changing …

Now my special friend is Beverley Bates. She has helped me a lot and helps me sort out my problems. Everything has changed a lot. I don't do handicrafts or out-work any more. I go to College sometimes and do shopping and type wage packets for Dot and help in a local home. I like to be kept busy. I also do the savings group. I bank it and when we get enough money we go out for a meal or visit somewhere.

During the last two years I have been doing college courses and typing and computers. Everything has changed a lot. I find it hard to cope with all the changes and people coming and going.

Emma used to make charts for me. If I did well I got a gold star. But if I did not do well I got a black spot. Emma and Kathy left to have a baby each. Now I have Nicky Page. She has helped me a lot. She talks to me and sorts out my problems. She sorts out my weekends. She also helped me with relaxation lessons.

Chapter 5 Special Olympics

One of the things I have enjoyed about the Centre is the sports. I have won lots of trophies and medals, for athletics, throwing the softball and darts. The one I remember well is just before Prince Charles got married. I was throwing the javelin and I got teased about missing Charles when I threw as we didn't want him to miss his wedding and another time we went to Liverpool and Princess Alexandra was there. The Red Arrows did a display and parachuted onto the Stadium.

I enjoy my spare-time activities such as going to clubs, The Gateway and Openway and the Centre Club. I also belong to the Society at Church where we perform once a year different shows. Our choir leader works us very hard and we usually mange to put on a good show.

I have been very lucky in my life. Mom and Dad look after me and I have two sisters and nieces and nephews and lots of good friends.

Her book finished when she was 35.

The episodes

Her childhood had always been marked by outbursts.

> 'When she was sharing a bedroom with a sister, we came in once or twice when she was throwing books and thrashing around and we wondered if this was a fit.'

It was decided that these were behavioural and she was given largactil from early childhood to 1992, nearly 30 years. Peggy did not think it helped much and the idea of epilepsy was not followed up. Later, at one adult centre, she had tried computers which may have precipitated a series of fits that were clearly epileptic.

> 'I had a pacemaker.'

He mother explained that after the fits the doctors found that her heart had stopped three times so they decided to put in a pacemaker.

> 'I had to go in a room. The doctor showed me the pacemaker and he talked to me all about the operation. The thing is here under chest.'

Peggy continued,

> 'Her Dad had a heart attack and did not have the chance of a pacemaker, so she decided to have it. Her fits began, maybe, in 1990 with stomach ache and gritting of her teeth and then a full fit. She had a scan and they put her on tablets. They were surprised that she was on largactil for her hyperactivity. Before the pacemaker, she would have to hang onto people when walking, after she felt confident enough to walk on her own.
> After the operation the doctor asked us go to a presentation with all the other doctors in rows sitting there with the epilepsy nurse. They had a chart with all the stuff on Möbius; they all asked questions and a lot did not know anything about it. I got some of the explanatory forms from the Moebius Support Group to take to hospital each time after that.'

The support group

It was not until Alison was 41 that they knew she had Möbius. The local paper had an article on a girl with Möbius, raising money for her to have smile surgery and Peggy realized that Alison also had it.

'We never knew anything before then. Nothing. They just told us she was mentally handicapped.'

They went to a conference of the Moebius Support Group and had a wonderful time, seeing others with the condition for the first time. Alison loved playing with the children. It was, Alison said, 'Like living in a bubble.'

Peggy said, 'It was wonderful and we made friends. Then we went to Manchester for a day with those with Möbius, trying a facial stimulator, though the doctor said not to use it because of her pacemaker. We really felt at home. At the open day there was a young lady with twins, one with Möbius and one without, and she asked me how I coped and I said I just treated her as normal. I really felt at home.' Alison too felt at ease. How often, I wondered, had she felt like that.

Whilst they were there, there was a wedding in the hotel. Alison said, 'I got all the sparkly bits and gave them to the girls.' She had collected all the confetti and given it to the children; Peggy found her surrounded by all the mess, having a wonderful time. 'She would make a very good supervisor for children.'

'Oh yes, I would sort them out. I do you sometimes. I have to remind you about things at times when you forget. At church, I light the candles, check the wine and do the altar, morning and night. As sidesman I give the books out. I go round with the plate. I enjoy that. If a sidesman cannot do it I fill in.'

She used to help with the cooking and shopping for the old people associated with the church, but now they have died off she takes the church magazines out and collects the money. Every Saturday afternoon she goes shopping for hours, talking to everyone in the charity shops.

Peggy added, 'I am really vexed. My husband died 12 years ago now; I wish we had gone to the conference earlier.'

Vacuum

I asked Alison if she could tell if people were happy or sad. 'Like what?' she asked. Peggy asked if Alison could tell if she was angry.

'Yes,' she replied, 'you go red.' She seemed less sure about the moods of strangers and changed the subject. 'When Dad died I had fits.'

Peggy continued,

'Since he died I have been in a vacuum, trying to cope with everything. He was very good with her. We would separate our time away; I would go to the Choral Society once per week and he would go out with his friends on another day. Alison used to go to weekend respite but that has closed … the last 10 years since Will died have been a bit fraught. She hates being ignored. Once in Church a friend ignored her and she hated this. 'I'll sort it out Alison, I'll sort it out,' I said. My eldest daughter says that will be on my tomb stone.'

Alison added:

'I get frustrated when there is no College or anything. I go shopping with my friends and have a cup of tea and go bowling usually on a Wednesday, but not today [because of my visit]. Friends from Day Centre, older ones and younger ones – they go to the Day Centre to give their parents a break. I used to climb out the window and run up the street. I wobble when I walk, maybe because of the eye sight. What else should we talk about now, Mum?'

Peggy asked how the Möbius affected her.

'The eyes. I can't see much from the left. I can read OK, but have to hold my eyelid up the whole time.'

I had seen a photo of Alison and her father sitting on a beach, when she was 4. He was holding up one of her eyelids. She still does this to see anything. Her mum said that eating was also a big problem.

'If we eat out I explain and ask people to be tolerant of the way she eats. I try to sit facing the world and have Alison facing a wall. She never notices and doesn't worry. If, on a bus, teenagers stare or taunt, I get upset but she ignores them.'

'At the day centre I did a raffle and made snakes, frogs, and cushions. Made things and raised £136.' For a holiday that in the end she did not go on. Peggy explained that Alison was helpful at the Centres but not at home. She continued,

'I can only go out when she is at the club. I don't like bingo or whatever. When there is a choral concert I get a carer in, but it is only once a year. I have nowhere to go. Church friends go to the club where they play bingo. There isn't anything that takes me. My daughters live away and one teaches. I go away with one of them, and my grandsons come every Thursday to see me. They used to come after school and now in their twenties they still come. I go out Tuesday night to Choral Society, when Alison goes to Mencap.

Peggy is wary of Alison having a fit without her being there, so she is reluctant to leave her, even with a carer. 'Her Dad and I used to alternate. The fits vary, every two or three months.'

Ptosis spectacles

'What else do you want to know?' Alison asked. I asked what she would like to be different.

'Be nice to have my eyes fixed. The right is worst, and I cannot see well out of it. I cannot move my eye sideways. I am worried the anaesthetic might set my fits off. I don't mind needles. I am going to the opticians to sort out my glasses.'

She had had special 'ptosis glasses' to try to stop the skin in her eye-lids falling down over the eyes. They were just ordinary glasses with small bars behind the lenses to hold up the skin. Despite waiting weeks for them to be made they did not work.

Her mother asked what it was like compared with her sisters who had grown up and married with children. Had she ever thought about that?

'It would be nice, to be included in what they do, playing games and that.'

Peggy replied,

'When we first came here there were fields at the back and the other girls and their Dad played in them, but Alison did not go out there; she played on the front where we could watch. The lady across the road would call her children in when she was out. It made you conscious of the disability. We may have been over protective, but she has done things her sisters have not, like the Special Olympics.'
'I enjoyed this, running, with the feet.'

Peggy asked,

'Did you ever wish to get married?
'No, not get married. I never wanted to get married.'

One long-term boyfriend had only communicated via the phone or valentines. I said that some people don't marry anyway. Peggy asked if being tied up with her was the problem.

'No, you are not boring. You are very patient. I like holidays, being in a jail.'

Once, during a tour of Durham Gaol she had needed the toilet and went into a jail cell by mistake. Peggy was surprised that Alison had not said more; they had been looking forward to my visit for some time. But Alison was not sure what to say, so Peggy continued.

> 'Her biggest problem is a frustration that she cannot say all that she wants to say, even though she talks non-stop. We've been so ignorant of so many things; there was no one to help. Even now, with Social Services, we never get any advice. We get no assistance at all. We just get on with it. We used to have a community nurse, but the only advice we got was put her into care for the weekend to give you a break. But Alison likes to go to Church on a Sunday and shopping Saturday and I didn't want to break that. Since my husband died she does go to respite when I go on holiday with my other daughters, and I take her on holiday once a year.
>
> 'She goes to a Day Centre Monday to Friday, apart from the Old People's Home on Thursday afternoon. Then there is the Mencap Club on Tuesday, Gateway club Monday night, once per month, Thursday Friends' Club, ring and ride. Saturday is cooking in the morning and shopping in the afternoon. Church on Sunday; while I cook, iron, clean, and keep her going.'

As funding becomes tighter some Centres are closing, reducing their options. Her present Centre is due to close. Even those kept open have fewer staff and facilities, so there is less to do, meaning more shopping or visits to garden centres.

> 'She does get bored; maybe gets bored with me.'
> 'I don't get bored with you.'

Peggy then fetched her own memoir. She had discussed everything with me, in front of Alison, with gentleness and humour. This changed as she read her diary.

> 'Oh, dear, it looks like we went through a lot of anger at the time. I have forgotten. It might be useful for you to read it. This sounds awful looking at it now. I had forgotten all this.'

It was started 17 years ago, in early 1988, though she began the account earlier.

Peggy's Memoirs

(Reproduced with permission)

5th January 1956

A cold foggy day at four o'clock in the afternoon; two little girls sitting on the stairs waiting the arrival of their new brother or sister. One was 7, the other 4. Alison arrived, no birth problems though it was noticed she had a very lopsided cry and swollen eyelids. The first words my mother said to my husband were, 'You couldn't do anything right.' She had wanted a boy. We were delighted.

Problems soon started; Alison wasn't able to feed properly. She hadn't opened her eyes. Our local doctor decided to send her to hospital and when she came home her eyes were partly open, but one eye turned out, rolling continually. My heart sank, as some years previously I had seen a baby like this who was mentally handicapped.

She was quite a good baby for a few months. When she walked at 17 months her Dad showed her how to hold up her eyelids to help her see. She started saying a few words and at 18 months old was admitted to the Eye Infirmary for surgery to one eyelid which was stitched back. She was in hospital for four weeks and was such a handful that a net was put over her cot to cage her in. She stopped talking. We visited every day.

She had two or three further operations and had regular visits for 12 years or so without much progress, apart from glasses. Then she was discharged as no more could be done.

To the present day she holds up her eyelids to see properly.

During her early childhood she was a handful, hating sitting in a pram or pushchair.

At 4 she was admitted on a day basis to a nursery because she was slow talking. At school age she had tests and was refused a normal school education. I had to keep her at home till she was 7, though a teacher came to help. No normal school would have her, since she was so overactive.

Keeping her occupied every day was quite a job; she would lock me out when I went to peg out the clothes, turn on the taps, and flood the kitchen. She would climb out the window to seek company …

She went to a number of schools and training centres and boarded during the week.

During times at home we would be awakened during the night with objects – books, toys, anything to hand, being thrown across the room. Alison moaned loudly and long, banged on walls and was quite uncontrollable. She would be sick and have fits.

When Alison was 8 she went to another boarding school with weekends at home. One school locked her in her bedroom at night; another would not have her back after a few weeks, citing behavioural problems. The local MP was kind and caring and arranged for her to go to a special day school. She stayed there till she was 16 when she left to go to a Training Centre, where she is to this day.

During her young years she had many fits, some severe; the doctor gave her largactil and tryptizol. [This medication was to calm her down and certainly not for epilepsy.] Sometimes she was quite violent and smashed door frames and windows. She has grabbed chair legs while we have been sitting in them and upended them – big arm chairs. During one outburst, in 1982 when she was 26, she was so bad that I could not handle her and had to call for a friend, the local vicar, and he stayed four hours while my husband came home from work. When she was violent it took two of us to hold her down.

The most trivial things upset Alison and she would react violently. If she was promised something and it didn't happen she went to pieces and flew into a rage. If not collected for a club, she would be uncontrollable for hours. We have kept so many incidents of violence to ourselves because we had no one to help or turn to. Our local doctor did not understand.

We tried to give our other girls as normal life as possible and they were very good with Alison. Both passed their exams and one is now a teacher; the other works for the government. We always tried to take the children to the seaside on holiday, usually in a caravan. We would come home exhausted.

We decided to try to get a break ourselves and found a holiday home at North Wales that would take mentally handicapped. We took her Friday to Friday and had a short break in between; she went there each summer for five years and then the home closed. After that she was placed in a home with some elderly patients. Despite apprehension by Mom she enjoyed 'looking after them' as they were less able than her. She asked when she could go again.

She is something of a Jekyll-and-Hyde personality, aggressive and argumentative at home and quite helpful and friendly to outsiders, so most people have no idea of the traumas she causes at home. She occasionally lets herself down though. One thing she hates is being ignored and when a friend of ours at church ignored her because she caught Alison giving me a thump, she yelled and cried in Church and had quite a tantrum. She mislaid a brooch she had been bought and knocked over the Christmas tree. If she mislays something it is hell until we find it; then she immediately forgets it.

If she gets upset with someone she will come home and tear at her hair and agitate me to 'sort it out'.

Days in which we do not have a problem are few and far between. How much longer can we cope? We are 60 and 63 now. Alison's answer to this is, 'You are not going to have me put away.' Where she gets this idea from I don't know.

She goes out Tuesdays to one club, Wednesdays to another and Thursdays to a third; the other nights she is miserable. She has her own portable TV, record player, cassette player, tapes, etc., and has lost interest in them all. If she is not interested in a TV programme there is no way she will let us watch it. To read a newspaper is a signal for her to vie for attention.

She hates any change in routine and rebels most strongly. Once she was due to go to a home for weekend respite. When she found her favourite warden was not on duty she asked if she might break her wrists so she could go another weekend.

This account only scratches the surface of 32 years. What of the future? We can't see it getting any easier.

December 1988, aged 32

21st December 1988

Very exhausting day, two weeks with elder daughter ill in hospital, going early to take their boy to school, work, visiting hospital, shopping for Christmas, and then pick up Alison, who was agitated that she might have to leave the centre. From 3.20 to 11.20 she has not let up. At one point exhausted, she lay down, so I started to watch a film; that was her chance to start again. I had to physically force her to bed and she refuses to get undressed. I'm going to have a drink and hopefully sleep.

27th December 1988

She wants some fun out of life – you've had yours she says – I wonder which day that was.

1989

I have to play guessing games with her. Conversations about small things resurface weeks later with no reference. I went with her to a barn dance. Alison did not enjoy it much. One man sat a yard away but did not talk [to us], so goodbye friend, enjoy your farewell speeches; I will not be there to listen.

At church she badgered a man having to close the youth club because of older children throwing fireworks and being a nuisance. There were tears and moans. She does not want to stay in the house while I am off gallivanting – 7 till 7.45 choir practice one day per week.

At one stage a psychologist was suggested, 'What have I got to see her for, I'm not mad.' Though reassured, she was agitated and ran upstairs and began to laugh like the madwoman in Jane Eyre.

I don't think anyone will ever understand her; I don't after 33 years.

Came back once and Alison was in tears. She had been asked to change to another room at the centre. She phoned the woman and said something but then was distressed and wrote to apologize after days of anxiety, 'Will Jenny understand, will she be angry?' We were almost demented.

Just to choose her coat or mac throws her into confusion. Some nights she runs up and down stairs laughing and yelling. Can Dr L sleep – we can't.

Friday, 14th. Really upset over an incident; she was told off at the Centre. She admits she had a tantrum but said that B had made her lose her crisp money in the machine. No reasoning with her. I rang for advice from a nurse; there was no one, so we had to suffer on.

Sister and brother-in-law came. In conversation he saw how Alison rules our lives. To outsiders, she is friendly and helpful; at home she gets so aggressive. Waiting for a letter, the postman passes by, she gets upset.

One night she asked the same questions again and again. I was tired and went to bed. She followed me so I slapped her legs and then I was upset.

I asked her next morning why she keeps on and on when a question is answered, 'You don't answer right.'

Some weeks where Alison has been quite settled, going to the Centre and each day's pattern is working well. We did our annual show in the Church Hall. She does very well, remembering all the words and music but she worries where to stand; everyone helps.

Went to the theatre by bus. Alison enjoys drawing attention to herself, talking loudly and pulling at her eyelids, making them sore. We had to move seats in the theatre since she was distracting those round her.

She started mithering her Dad about not going to Church. Saying that he does not want to any more is not enough. She goes on for hours and hours and then goes berserk and kicks in a door panel, swearing. It is like living with a time bomb.

When Will had an accident the car was damaged and so he had to walk Alison to various evening activities, wait three hours and then walk her back, despite being soaked on the way.

At one stage she wanted to go on holiday and talked of burning down the hostel and the mentally handicapped there; in her words there will be less of 'them' to look after and feed. I'm at my wits end; she goes on non-stop; putting up with it is bad enough at home but to go amongst other people and listen to her onslaughts I could not bear. I got so embarrassed by her behaviour. When I ask her to be quiet she says, 'I don't care about those bastards …' I looked around and most parents and children were behaving well. I find conversing with anyone impossible; Alison just butts in and takes over.

She is a mass of contradictions, hating the Centre and yet not wanting to leave. Halfway back from her sister's for Christmas [a car journey] she went to the toilet and ran off for half an hour into a funfair.

Bit put out when she came home from resident's home; they cheered as she left.

I could not have a phone conversation because she always takes it over. She got angry because I wanted to go to bed rather than watch TV late at night. I went to bed and ignored her in the end.

Had a right tantrum at the Centre when someone threw away a small amount of milk which she usually drinks. Moaned for two hours after we got home. Next morning she apologizes as usual, so she knows she is playing up.

August holiday here again. two weeks for me at home whilst she is at the Centre.

Decided not to go to daughter's for Christmas; Alison demands too much attention and resents any I give to anyone else.

She treats me like we have a yard of elastic between us. Everywhere I go she follows; if I speak she wants to know what it is I'm talking about.

Sunday dinner an hour late and she moaned … she wanted it at the right time. The Christmas Party was cancelled because of snow and lack of transport, so she walked there anyway. She came back soaked but at least she realized everything had stopped.

1991

Christmas was calm; Alison did not have to share attention with anyone. As January is progressing though she appears bored with parents and after her 35th birthday party a difficult period.

Monday. Alison gone to Home, Will to bowls, dejected I do the ironing.

Couldn't find umbrella, for four hours she was demented, she would not shut up about the most 'treasured present'. We feel so down in the dumps and at a loss to cope. Umbrella found in knitting bag next day.

Finding something for her to fill in time is becoming more difficult, she has finished most of the courses. There was an open day at the Centre and she was very proud of the things she had done and was very helpful. A beetle drive at Church, she was awful because she did not win. I did and got a real earbashing.

Weekends are difficult because there is little for her to do. One day she was a body at a swimming pool lifesaving. She is so demanding that we are finding it more difficult to cope. All we get are continuous verbal attacks. She is selfish and not interested in anything we want to see.

I could just throw her out of my sights, she makes us so unhappy. The vicar is leaving Monday; she never liked him but now is upset he is going.

April 1992

Easter; no clubs, tearing at clothes and generally going berserk. Saturday she went to an Easter Bonnet party and won £10, Sunday she went to a party ... her social life is much better than ours – we are here to cope with her demands.

Will died 25th September 1993, traumatic time.

The diary ends New Year, 1994.

Many fits and incontinence at Church Hall. Realized that A's naughtiness is epileptic fits not being treated ... we have all suffered unnecessarily.

Since she hardly picks up expressions and moods in others, her own lack of facial expression has not been a problem for Alison. Her face problems are mainly to do with eating and drinking, and, of course, because to see she has to hold up the lid of her one good eye.[4]

Learning difficulties and autism are often considered problems of the young. But children become adolescents and then adults and, though less evident to society, their problems may persist. Peggy is now in her late seventies and Alison is in her early fifties. Möbius syndrome is not just about the face; Alison's problems have been with learning difficulties and social interaction, each made difficult by the ptosis. Many of her problems have fallen on her family; to her sisters, growing up with such a demanding sister, and to her parents, bringing her up with their other two daughters. Now, in her seventies, the burden is Peggy's alone.

Chapter 8

Hear my smile

One of them

Matthew Joffe is a prominent elder statesman within the US Moebius Syndrome Foundation, much respected and admired for his work and – perhaps even more – for his example within the community. We sat one hot New York day in a hotel lobby in the lower East Side.[1]

'My grandmother was peering over at me in my crib and I remember a sort of mobile hanging, arching out, over my head. I remember the wallpaper because I asked my Mum later about it and she said I must have been about 6 months of age where we lived at that time. At 2 years of age I remember houses with steps up from the street and then a landing and steps into the house, in Queens, and I remember being in a stroller and it was a lovely day with lots of foliage on the trees and I was just being wheeled down the street. I also remember swimming in Southampton, Long Island, because my parents had a place we went each summer and I remember learning to swim at 2.

'I was born on 60th and 3rd in Leroy's Sanatorium. One day I saw the sign still there past Bloomingdale's. I lived in Jackson Heights for the first four years and I remember bouncing up and down on my parents' bed. Then we moved to Long Island and I lived there till I was 18 and went to college. I went to grad school in NYC and have lived there ever since.

'I studied psychology and French and was very fortunate to have a teacher who was an authority on psychology. He was a legend; and you either liked him or loathed him. I thought his the worst class I had ever been in. Then something happened; by the middle of the semester everyone in the class loathed him except me. One day he put out a challenge. He said that no one could get an A in his class unless they did a paper. The exams were not enough. He threw out an idea about a 17th century Frenchman who may have been the first to coin the word 'psychology'. He wanted someone to translate a paper of his. The idea intrigued me and I went up to him. From that moment on I had my own mentor. He took me under his wing and for an hour at a time we would discuss translation. It was like the tutorial system at Oxford and Cambridge; I felt so honoured. It helped me to know what it was to give something back to others – a life-shaping experience.'

Matthew went to Lehigh, an engineering school in Bethlehem, Pennsylvania, which had some business and liberal arts as well. In a nice area, it also had a good reputation for social life, and he was not looking for somewhere without a social life. It was also close enough to go home for the weekend.

> 'These years were truly special. I have always loved languages; they are the key to understanding another country's soul. I studied French in High School and was not going to stop. I knew when I was 16 what I wanted to do. I was very clear and focused; as for psychology, I wanted to help people and talk to them about their problems.'

He enrolled in a psychologist doctoral programme, but the competitive atmosphere did not suit. Instead he went into a training programme to be a therapist and analyst after his teaching programme at Columbia. He has no regrets about not completing his doctorate. Now he directs the Office for Students with Disabilities at LaGuardia College, part of the City University of New York (CUNY), in Queens. He is also an educational/learning disability therapist, and does diagnostic work including ADD, ADHD, and Asperger's syndrome, and with people with psychological disorders.

Enrolment at the school is traditionally at 18 but since they also serve a large number of non-traditional populations, there are all ages and cultures represented. Matthew soon learned that different cultures view disability differently.

> 'For instance, in some cultures there is a notion of shame if a family has a disability. Or, they may view an assessment as a threat. We have to help them understand other ways of viewing disability. When working with a student, one has little access to their family, which may be living in their original country's thought patterns. Students can have opposite messages at home and school. Having to choose between cultures may not be easy.
>
> 'Those with Asperger's can have a problem with faces, interpreting clues. I do not know what they see when they talk with me; I can only say I am accepted. I get the sense that when they talk, I am one of them ... My students with Asperger's look me in the eyes.'

The booby prize

From round 18 months he had difficulties holding his head up and his mouth began to droop. His mother used to massage his cheek to help him chew. He was diagnosed at 4. After lots of tests, including one involving an injection to exclude myasthenia gravis, they said that, by default, he had, 'The booby prize, Möbius.' His parents anguished about the injection since he was so scared by it; he was haunted by it for years.[2]

> 'Years later they took me into an old Columbian Presbyterian Hospital room with an old frosted glass and a wooden door. They are drawing blood like I was a specimen, and this is 1957 now, and the next thing I know they tapped my carotid and I remember screaming my head off. My parents were down the hall. At that time I developed an awful, deep-rooted dread of having my blood taken. Injections are fine, but the moment they want to take blood I sweat buckets. I screamed and cried and panicked.'

When he was 12, playing in a yard, someone slapped him in the face and his mouth closed. They all just stood there in amazement. The doctors thought it was too much calcium. Waiting for a blood test, he sat next to a 6-year-old kid who was calm while he was a 'basket case', shaking and sweating. At the time he did not know what it was about since he had blocked the original memory.

Then, sitting at home as a teenager, he saw a hospital newsletter article about a doctor being given a new position and saw this man and said, 'Holy Shit, it was him.' He was head of the team who had taken blood from his carotid and he realized why he dreaded having blood taken. Once he understood he began to come to terms with it. At 16 he had done his own analysis.

> 'Eventually I could control blood-taking procedures. I walk in and say here are the ground rules; my way or no blood, no discussion. I insist on a butterfly needle in the right hand. Once it got to the surface I understood it. It was grist to the mill of my becoming a therapist.
>
> 'I hold the medical profession in this country in great contempt. They have never taken the time to learn how to talk to and listen to people and to take a patient as being more than the sum of their problems. It is this that I rail against with great ferocity. For years I would give them a hard time and be very sarcastic, sometimes even caustic, which is why I am so fond of English humour. I loved my paediatrician but I went to various specialists and was disappointed by their inability to follow through on what they said and by their lack of empathy.'

His eyes have always been a problem and have deteriorated over time. He has always needed glasses. Without much blink, he has had exposure keratitis. In 1993 and 1999 he had gold weights placed in the upper lids and his lower ones were lifted and sutured. 'Actually they blinded me in one eye; the closure of the eye limited its usefulness. They closed the eye to protect the cornea since I am not a transplant-eligible individual.' He has no peripheral vision to the right, glaucoma and chronic conjunctivitis with great sensitivity to sunlight. He lives in wide-brimmed hats and dark glasses. 'I have had surgery on my eyes six times and have quarterly check-ups. Doctors like to watch it.'

He has chronic problems with teeth too. He had several removed by a dentist as a child, leading to a lifetime of dislike of the profession. He also was very sensitive and has had bouts of trigeminal neuralgia. Eager to inform, he still goes once a year to the University of Medicine and Dentistry of New Jersey, where he helps teach dental students about treating people with disabilities.

> 'I have always had to cut my food into small pieces. I bob my head when eating to gain momentum and power in chewing, partly because of my neck problem. I cannot hold my head up long because it hurts. I eat red meat less because it takes so much chewing and I can get trigeminal neuralgia. I prefer my bread toasted because it is easier to eat. I never eat corn on the cob or ribs in public; I don't do horizontal eating because I make a mess and so I do it at home only.'

He was also angry with doctors for not making his Möbius go away. Every hospital visit he left without anything, at least in his own mind. His other concern was the lack of awareness of patient's feelings by doctors. His poem 'Doctor, Doctor' is about this.

'Doctor, Doctor'

Doctor, Doctor, 'What's the matter with me?'
Out in the real world, I can only see
the faceless eyes, staring back at me!

I feel like a movie star surrounded by white
the language is foreign the quarters are tight
the project begins the voices swell to a din
Hey wait! Wait for me, I've committed no sin!

Often I look back and see danger lurking around me
A curio mounted and displayed for all to see
by residents, doctors, nurses – onlookers no doubt
so lonely uninformed incapable of figuring it out.

For years my life was defined by what you see
I'm guilty as much for contributing to me.
No more do I want to be someone's discovery.

A word! A touch! A smile! A glance!
Could it be that hard? Come on take a chance
towards hope and dignity and life at the brim
Just once drop your facade – go out on a limb.

Discover an answer, a chance to understand
why my eyelid hangs loosely, why I've got one good hand
Doctor, Doctor, 'Can't you open your book
find me a cure, give me back what they took!'

Reproduced by permission

This was written only nine years ago, when Matthew was 41. He had raged for a long time against doctors. Only then, in his forties, did he no longer hold them responsible.

The 59th Street Bridge

He had surgery at age 4 for tonsillitis and woke up during the operation, remembering bright lights and a doctor panicking, 'Oh my God, he's awake.' Later in a room at the end of a long corridor, his mother must have gone for a cup of coffee as he slept. He woke to find his mother gone and was terrified. He was unable to scream because of the operation; a nurse came eventually.

'I had a primal feeling of abandonment. I have coped with it my whole life; it is very important for me to have my apartment, for instance, feel very much lived in and an extension of me and a safe place. It is important to maintain contact with people. This feeling of being alone has stayed.

'If I sit in my apartment late at night and look out I feel alone. It is the one aspect of New York that still haunts me, and I am a big fan of New York. It is the one part of my life that I sometimes worry about and certainly contemplate; being alone. I have lots of good friends but I don't have my own intimate relationship with a woman. As people get married and have children they drift away. Being alone in the city is still there. It is not raw and it is not fresh but it is still alive.'

For some with Möbius early childhood is a kind of Eden, socially at least, when, within family and close young friends, they are hardly aware of their visible difference (though many of the more physical problems are there). Later when cliques form at school, or during adolescence and beyond, these become more evident. But Matthew did not remember things that way. His problems began early, aged 4 or 5 with name calling and ridicule.

'I was very isolated at school. I would go to school and then come home and do my homework and the day was weighing on me. Later, I was not allowed to drive, so I was dependent on my Mom. Those years in particular I would like to do different, looking back.'

Struggling with his peers, he gravitated towards adults. Even now he is more comfortable around adults.

'However well adjusted you are, if you go to a friend's house and a child turns to his mum and says, "He looks funny," I would be lying if I said it does not hurt at some level. I can deal with it, have been dealing with it all my life, but it does not mean I do not feel it inside.'

Junior High was hard and isolating too.

'One thing came out of it. One day I was having lunch with a friend. He went out and was jumped on by three people for having lunch with me. He fought back and was brought to the principal. I said I would be his Perry Mason.

'I went to the Principal, in his late forties, and said that, though I didn't condone the violence and fighting, I didn't think it was fair that he should be punished for choosing me as his friend. I was 13 or 14. He thanked me for coming and for my loyalty to my friend and promised he would not suspend him. I walked out and realized that (a) I was a survivor and (b) I could stand up for myself. Those two things I have taken through my life, they made my sense of self.'

'Stepping out'

The prism of people glitters as
the potpourri of faces breeze by me.
There are all kinds of beautiful people
I too want to feel the breeze.

A celebration beyond the haves and have-nots,
pity stems from those who have nothing else to give.
The remains of my own frost melted quickly
reminiscing to music – nostalgia without the tears.

Stepping out this time meant stepping in
Schmoozing with someone whose hand touches yours
and whose aura says welcome.
All of a sudden you forget the fears.

I am learning to be vulnerable in public –
pride without excuses.
My heart vibrates with the beat of the sun.
The warmth of others lets the breeze fall on my face.

Reproduced with permission

My own voice

'My friends were doing alcohol and drugs when it was the rage in the 1960s and the Vietnam War. I refused. My high in life will be natural. I was saying that even with all my problems I would not take drugs, and this and my disability threatened them and their choices to drink and try marihuana and LSD. I was not going to be anything but my own man.

'My parents always, always, always told me that when I was being teased it was not about me but the other person. This became larger and larger in my mind and contributed to my sense of self.

'Of all the things done to improve me, the single most important was speech therapy. I began aged 5 and continued until I was in junior high. I had so much I thought all kids had it. Winding down with my therapist at the end of the summer term in ninth grade, I asked who was going to be my therapist the next year. She looked at me, smiled, and said I was not going to have one. I felt like lying on the table and crying out, 'What do you mean I am not going to have any more?' They gave me the ability, literally, figuratively, and spiritually, to find my own voice.

'When I was born my mouth was down where my jaw is now and I spoke in a very low guttural voice. They taught me to bring my voice forward to speak clearly and to not speak and swallow. I still remember what I sounded like at aged 4; only my parents and a few others could understand me. Some even thought I was contagious; if we played tag they did not want me to be "it", in case they caught Möbius. This was very hurtful.

'The speech therapy was revolutionary. It opened up so much, and not just speech. I became a thinker. I have always been pensive rather than extroverted. I am not athletic. My weapons and tools are words and communication. They form a large part of my sense of self, and of my conviction that, despite all the problems of Möbius, I have always believed that no one and nothing is going to stop me from leading my life. Whilst I have had to make some radical changes in my life habits I refuse to throw in the towel. I am going out kicking and screaming and doing what I want to do till the very end.

'The other part of my sense of self is my sense of humour. When I meet someone without a sense of humour I cannot communicate with them.'

Wittgenstein wrote that humour is not a mood but a way of looking at the world.[3] Matthew agreed that it is your perspective on life that makes things funny. 'When I was 8, I had to have two injections in the leg, one white and one orange liquid. The nurse decides to put both into the same syringe and gives the mixture to one site. She says, "Isn't that cool?" All of a sudden it starts to come out and drip onto the sheet. I say to her, aged 8, "You proud of this? Now clean it up and get out." He laughed.

Listen carefully ...

'I guess I can honestly say that if I had my time over, I would spend more time developing hobbies I could do alone rather than being focused on trying to find playmates. I guess I was lonely and missed an opportunity to develop things to do by myself.'

Earlier that day I had just walked past a New Yorker with a T-shirt slogan, 'Do I look like a people person?' Not every one is, of course, but they have an element of choice.

'I did not have choice in the eyes of others. But from day one I knew what I wanted to do with my life professionally, and it was always contact with others, helping them. I never wanted an office job; I am a people person. The struggle is to get others to see it like that. Our plays [Matthew writes and acts in plays as part of a support group, Inner Faces (supported by Forward Face), which has an acting troupe within it] are telling people, "Look at us, look beyond the face. Who's more disabled; those who discriminate, or us?"'

Nicola Rumsey, a professor of Health Psychology at the University of the West of England has carried out some research on the self-confidence of those with cleft palate during adolescence. To her surprise, they found that people with cleft actually had more confidence than their control subjects without any condition.[4] Those with cleft had been forced to come to terms with these concerns earlier and more deeply than others. Matthew agreed and thought that he had done the same.

'I express my emotions. I have wide range of laughs for different experiences and I use them for where my facial expression does not go. I also play with ways of speech and inflections of voice. If I ever wrote about my life, my title would be *If You Listen Carefully, You Can Hear Me Smile*. I use all these things to overcome the lack of facial expression. I have never wanted to play poker or be a ventriloquist. I knew at a subconscious level that there were limits to my expressiveness and I must have come up with ways to overcome it – since none of this is taught – for as long as I can remember.

'Working with Paul Ekman[5] I had to look at faces and then describe them, and I found that so frustrating. I don't look at people that way because I cannot give out expressions. If someone says something about someone else, then I would find it hard to describe his or her features. It is also difficult to describe facial expressions; how do you make a frown? I can't, so it's hard.[6]

'I communicate my moods in my voice without my smile, by jumping up and down and in talking faster than I normally would. When I won an award at the university, I called people up and said, "I WON!" I do it like others, except for the smile. People can really see my mood. I sometimes say my moods. People who know me know if I am sad, or unhappy or annoyed because I won't speak. I'll sit there and I've been told my silences are deafening. I carry my body differently; it is weighted down when I am sad. I tend to withdraw and become introverted. Then I am more an observer than a participant, but this is not about the face. The face is about them, if you get the difference. The face expresses but does not define. The face does not define my sense of being.'

The way it is

The face does not define, I agreed, once people got to know someone, but Matthew had to manage new people each day, with visible difference. How does he manage this?

'The only honest answer is that you spend your entire life doing that. There is no point in time when you close the book and say that is over. It is a work in progress. I have made enormous strides in the way I handle the reactions of other people. Each time I walk on the street I have the potential to encounter this.

'When people look at me they are not necessarily clear about what they are seeing. There is a sort of caste system of disability about what is acceptable. If you see someone in a wheelchair you can draw some deductions; road accident, spinal injury, polio, but if you look at someone like me you are puzzled. I am aware of that. One of my reasons for the plays and Moebius support group and Inner Faces is to make people with craniofacial disabilities a larger part of mainstream lives, more a part of people's lives and social fabric. In Toronto, no one stared at me and I came back wishing that Manhattan had been like this. I have to put up with it; it is part of my life.'

Years ago, a friend of his at college, late one night, had confessed that it had taken him a while to get used to Matthew. Since it was a hard thing for a 20-year-old to say, he appreciated it. It helped him understand that it is a process for others which takes time. 'A Kodak moment.' To this day, when he does a workshop, he'll say. 'I'll tell you a secret. I know you think I look funny. It's OK cos that's the way it is.'

There was an attractive idea initiated some years ago about stage theory. After certain events, illness and injury, say, one had stages of reaction;

denial, anger, acceptance, etc. While this may be the case for some, for many it is not. In discussing reactions to becoming paraplegic with me once, Mike Oliver, a retired professor of disability studies and himself tetraplegic, refuted stage theory, suggesting adaptation was an endless continuing process. Matthew agreed. 'I agree with him. This challenge will follow me round all my life.'

I mentioned Albert Bull, a man made paraplegic during the Second World War. Lying in Stoke Mandeville Hospital, in England, he had said that the most important thing for a tetraplegic was to cheer up his visitors. Matthew was surprised but delighted.

> 'That's very profound and relates to my use of humour, absolutely. I don't want you feeling sorry for me, since my life may have been better than yours.'[7]

Zits and the Sistine Chapel

For a long time, Matthew avoided groups. Dances at junior high were terrible, High school was a black hole, in fact all his group experiences were a disaster. Then a couple of years ago he was participating with other Inner Faces members in a project at a school on Long Island and something earth-shattering happened. They had been taking classes on disability awareness all week. There was a girl who had sat in the back of the class and had said nothing. Then she asked to come again and when she did she sat next to Matthew. Just as they started, she burst into tears.

> 'The only way I can describe it – and it was very powerful for me – is like that great scene in the Sistine Chapel with God and Adam and the fingers and the thunderbolt of lightning between them. I felt this enormous electrical charge come out of her and land in me. It spoke to the absolute core of what it means to make contact with another person in the most profound way imaginable. She said that all she was worrying about were her zits and whether her boyfriend would take her out Saturday night and whether she would be liked. She felt after listening to us that all her issues were small and inconsequential. That initial electrical and chemical moment of connection I will take to my grave.
>
> 'Now I have experienced it, there is a part of me that is searching to have it again. It was such a tremendous experience and it took away all this superficial physical stuff and it said, "Society, get out of the way!" It was all about two human beings. If not the most powerful experience I have ever had, it is certainly in the top three. It took my breath away.'

'My own personal earthquake'

He went on to describe his first meeting with other people with Möbius, when he was aged 41. It was in Los Angeles in July, 1994.

'I walked into the hotel and there were 102 people standing there, either an adult with a child with Möbius, or they had Möbius.

'It was like having my own personal earthquake; a whole community, feeling we were all from the same place, all connected. It was fabulous. Parents said how much they have got from listening to me. I'm mature and have considered myself fairly wise, and parents seemed inspired, with, and not in spite of, Möbius. I got so much out of it, I have not missed a meeting since. I am presently Vice-President of the Foundation in the USA. I met a family I never knew. I had finally arrived at a place and a space that was mine. I could relate to individuals in a way I had never been allowed to anywhere else. Just to see other adults with it and just to have adults who wanted me around because their child had the same thing, rather than have me a painful reminder of their own situation.[8]

'It's important that you find your own voice. You need to find your own identity, your own person who happens to have Möbius but that does not mean you can't travel on your own road. My quest, my desire has been to be in the world, to do things because I want to and not because I get permission from others.

'I am living proof of having both Möbius and a quality of life and not settling for less because it's the only offer. Life is about what you do with it, in so many different ways.'

The attic

Within the UK Moebius Support Group there had been, until recently, only one married man. Others had talked of their problems with the first kiss and Matthew had spoken of the nightmare of the high school prom.

'Now you are approaching the attic. I have described my life as being like a house with many floors and rooms, and the attic is the only one without a light on; the romance one. It is the topic I hesitate to talk about the most.

'I was always questioning my ability to kiss properly, watching others do what they do. I give wet kisses and people will dry themselves off afterwards, and I feel guilty and self-conscious.

'I never had a girlfriend in high school. I never talked to a girl until I got to college, in all honesty. I never dated until I was older. I joined dating agencies and that did not work out. I even joined a classical music lovers' exchange, thinking that people who listen to classical music must be in some way elevated above the rest. I found out, in the harshest of ways, they can be just as unsavoury as anyone else.

'I was set up with a woman and we dated for round 6 months. She died unfortunately; she was one of the founding members of Inner Faces.'

Sometimes

Sometimes the words are there
and they're all I have to keep me from the ghosts of fantasy
Stepping outside my skin just once
risking all to taste the exquisite pleasure and pain

Sometimes the words are not enough
and I recoil in the shadow of my thoughts
How I yearn to tear through the fibers of my heart
and flood your soul with the waves of my tears

Sometimes I quietly cry myself to forget
what seems just around the corner
It is cold and I long for your touch
to help me warm my dreams

Sometimes I am alone and frozen
the words have left me unborn
I writhe amongst the ashes of passion
and wish I could surrender to the flames

Reproduced with permission

'The hardest thing for me to do in my whole life is to take the risk of being physical with a woman. It is something I have talked myself into doing, I know all the intellectual stuff and yet I find myself as though in cement shoes with my hands tied behind my back, unable to move and terribly afraid of the rejection I suffered as a child. The teasing and ridicule I suffered then was done mostly by boys. Yet I am – terrified is not strong enough a word – petrified of the fear of being rejected as an adult by a woman, and feeling incredibly insecure about technique and what is step 1 and step 2 and feeling horribly inexperienced and unworldly in those areas compared with others.

'Between dates there would be a tremendously long rebound period since I was so wounded and so frightened. I went to therapy and it has played a huge role in allowing me to see that my life was not defined, just as you – not personally – were implying by my inability to a smile, my life is not defined by whether I am married or with a woman.

'I have had a long journey and a rediscovery of what it means to be a masculine individual. With men, at least, I feel my disability maleness is different and/or jeopardized or traumatized as a result of the disability. A real man drove a car, a real man could be a stock boy in the summer earning money, a real man could put a nail in a wall with a hammer, all the things I could not do. Therapy helped me to hammer and chip and chisel away at it, so I have redefined who I am and what I can offer myself and the world and, if it is not for a relationship, I can enjoy my work with the plays and the documentaries, the music, my friends – my close friends who I have a lot of. If someone chose to be my friend it was a deep-rooted commitment for life.

'It does not mean I still don't desire it, but I acknowledge that perhaps, perhaps, the wound is so deep that I cannot overcome it. In one group therapy session one other member said that in a family fire, two out of three children were killed and he said that whatever anyone says the parents are never going to get over it. That stuck with me and gave me some sort of solace saying to myself that not everything can be surmounted. Just as Christopher Reeve, with all his research and notoriety, talked of walking again, part of me applauded his optimism and the other part thought of denial and the message he was giving out. There are things you just can't do. Maybe for me I can't get over this enormous fear of connecting physically with a woman and not having her spurn me. I am 50 years old and would basically start out as a high school kid. The woman for me is someone who is experienced and is willing to be a teacher. That is the way I would feel safest and most accepted, allowing me to blossom.'

I mentioned that, maybe, as we become older the physical part of a relationship reduced in importance, to be replaced by affection …

'It is interesting you say that. I talked with a friend at graduate school, saying everyone wants to have sex, and I would certainly like to have sex and know what that is like. At the same time, I said to him, that what I wanted more than anything else, I just want someone to hold me. I want someone to embrace me, to accept me, to love me; that is what really matters. There's all sorts of other stuff related to the physicality, which is designed to take place over time and which you learn to satisfy your partner and that stuff I just do not have a clue about – you need practise and I have had none, except by myself. It is so multilayered and complex.'

A palette of feelings

When he enrolled to become a certified psychotherapist and psycho-analysis, a condition of the course was that he was analysed. He said to the analyst, 'Let's get real; I know I could benefit from this. I am not just doing this for the course.' I always knew it would be helpful. 'It was a great experience; it taught me I could get in touch with my feelings, be angry and not be toxic.' Previously he was afraid to show feelings, afraid at how people would react. After all he had been attacked just for being.

'Anger was angst, focused on the condition and on a disability which made it tough as a 20-year-old kid to get on socially. I wanted to break out. All those things which typical, and not so typical, which were germane to being disabled.'

Several people with Möbius have said that they had difficulties in measuring how much emotion to show and to experience. They were afraid to be out of control of emotions and had difficulties in calibrating emotion against others. Matthew agreed.

'Yes, I may be suppressed. I was afraid because it might be a tidal wave, a volcanic, tirade, once I started I could not stop. I did not want to let the beast out of the cage. Therapy allowed me to get in touch with the palette of my feelings. It allowed me to explore the high spots, and the not so high, and it allowed me to take more risks, in employment, in speaking out, in assertiveness, talking from a position of emotions and not just intellect. Therapy was so influential and helpful.'

He is a therapist still. Along with alcohol and substance abuse therapy, family mediation and special education skills produce 'an interesting gestalt'. Everything he has done he uses, all are 'ingredients in the stew'.

'Each day I meet and work with someone, I see how an individual puts their stamp on a feeling. Each person is different and we all learn from each other. Everyone is on a journey; it is not about the life, it is about the journey. It is about what you did in that life and what you achieved. What decisions did you make and what did you learn.'

One of my teachers

'People always ask who would I want to be, and my answer is always the same; I don't want to be anyone but me. I like being me, with all that Möbius syndrome has brought into my life. I am no longer a Möbius syndrome individual; I am an individual with Möbius syndrome. Same words, but a different order and a whole new way of understanding what life is, and what the importance of life is even with a disability.'

'Given the choice'

Neither one of us is comfortable when we meet
If only our eyes met and we took the time
Instead, you make me laugh reminding me of my youth
turning the other cheek committing acts of contrition
where schoolkids ogled
and danced the dance of repugnance
I wish those days were behind me

In a lot of ways, I wish I looked like you
pumped up, tensile, blending right in

What price veneer?
I'm not sure of your values
nor how bright the light is inside
The truth is it is I who yearns to hit the dance floor
to sweat the venom projected upon me

I am making the choice for both of us
though only I will know its meaning
You've got what it takes
those other second looks that I covet
But what then – what comes after the gloss?
The echo confirms the emptiness that creeps out over your shadow
Given the choice, I'd rather be me

Reproduced with permission

'I joined the Inner Faces on 24 January 1994. I tell people that I have a tattoo inside on my heart with that date. There was a blizzard here in New York, so I went in my Cossack outfit.'

The support group was very important. As much as therapy prepared him for the world, being in a group where everyone had a common thread enabled him to feel he could stand on his own two feet. When he first joined the group he had been considering leaving his first job after 17 years, but knew it was not going to be easy, with a disability, to find another job. In the end he made the leap, had one interview and got the job.

'In my heart I know the cause of my empowerment and awakening was seeing myself differently, through the eyes of the group.'

'At the top of my voice I can now shout, like Peter Finch in Network, "I am mad as Hell, and I am not going to take it anymore." I want to feel contentment, pride, and feel that I was honest with myself and looked myself in the mirror. I want to be able to say that I have lived my life according to my mores and principles and did what I wanted to do.

'When I look in the mirror I see my body, absolutely, honestly. When I was 8, I was in the bathroom staring in the mirror and Mom was cleaning and I said, "You know, Mum, some people's faces are works of art; mine is Op Art." She just burst into hysterics and I was laughing. I see me there, the me that I know others do not see unless they get past the outside. What I see is mine; it does not belong to anyone else. It is part of who I am. It does not define, that's the stuff I see underneath and what I want so many others to see and get beyond this.

'In college, guys, and occasionally girls, would come to me with their boyfriend, girlfriend problems, and want me to give them advice. I was fascinated because I couldn't get a first date, let alone laid. Why me? I could not offer advice about technique or fore play and intercourse – sad but true – and yet they came to me. They did not see me as a sexual being and I was therefore safe to talk to about their sexual problem, which I did not appreciate.'

Like a celibate priest.

'And secondly, I would not judge them. I work hard to downplay the face, trying to make my personality clearly seen, not larger than life since that is a turn-off, but to make them realize there is more to me than my face.' In one of his documentaries, *Face: A Portrait*, Matthew wrote, 'To be with me is to be with my face.'

> 'You can't have me without my face since it is part of me. It is a statement and a challenge and call to embrace.
>
> 'The question of suicide is a real one. I knew two men with Möbius who committed suicide. It is such a loss. It is a painful and real issue and should be addressed further. Not just in Möbius but amongst the whole disability population. Not just because the risk may be higher but also because there might be signs. I don't think that anyone with Möbius has a stronger desire to know death than anyone else, but I felt more vulnerable. I could not discuss it with my other friends, though as we reach 50 the playing field might now be levelled. Why this should occur more in early adult life is a complex question. For some it may be the challenge to deal with their disability, to accept their reactions to rejection, disappointment with the struggle.'

Matthew's parents were told that he should not be a priority in their lives because he would be dead in a year. They fought for him in many ways, though it was not perfect. To balance protection from prejudice as best they could whilst giving him some resilience and confidence must have been so difficult. Then, at some point, they had to let him go. When he went to college, his mother felt the separation acutely. In contrast, his father, seeing him talking with the other students, was just relieved that he would make it on his own.

In their early years of junior high, his sister, after a friend had made fun of her having a disabled brother, had come running to their mother to ask if she would have to take care of Matthew when they were gone. Their Mom said no, if he had to he would take care of her.

> 'That was terrific since my mother saw me as a survivor. That bolstered my confidence. That's not to say there is not always something new to learn; perhaps one could say disability is one of my teachers.

'I was in Chicago on the South Shore, near the Aquarium and Soldier's Field, sitting in the sun with a hat and a book. There were boats on the lake and a couple a hundred yards away necking and I just sat there for two hours and it was absolute heaven. I could do that every day of my life and be as happy as can be. Water is very important to me. I have a picture by Andrew Wyeth of a rosebush over the sea because it reminds me of where I want to be. I am a great Wyeth fan. I also have *Christina's World*; she was a polio victim and walked with crutches or used a wheelchair, but in that picture she is normal looking.'

With many others, Matthew has been working within the Moebius Foundation to assist those with the condition. His life, he has decided, is not just for him. But he has also gone further; in several TV documentaries, and in his work with Inner Faces, Matthew has opened his experience to many.

'Originally, I was quite uncomfortable with being viewed as a role model. I struggled to see myself as others perceived me. I was uncertain how I would handle the responsibility. My head was turned in other directions, desperately trying to reconcile my place in the world, a world I had created, reflecting my own uneasiness with my own disability. Now, I wear my disability proudly. I have come full circle: instead of running from the eyes cast upon me, I look them straight in the eye. Only then can true acceptance, on both sides, be achieved.'

Chapter 9

'Doomed to express'

Berlin

Out of the blue, I was invited to talk at an international conference in Berlin, run by, and for, medical students. The invitation was flattering, mentioning that there were also lectures by Nobel Laureates. They asked if, in addition to a talk, I might comment as an artist drew a patient in front of a small crowd of students. In view of my interest in faces and in portraiture, this seemed too good to miss. Then, once I was hooked, they asked me if I could bring the patient over myself too and, ideally, that he or she would have a facial visible difference, to allow discussion of the face and its relation to the self.

I was very wary. Was it fair to expose someone with a facial disfigurement to such a process? After all, the students, and the artist, would focus on the face and might not look beyond it to the person beyond. But, in the end, I asked Henrietta. Being without facial expression, I reasoned, she would show them the limitations of taking a single visible image of a person. I was not sure Henrietta would agree, since it would take courage to expose one's face to a group of students who had probably never been exposed to facial differences. We had not met the artist, either; how would he react?

Henrietta thought for a while and then agreed. The chance to see Berlin may have helped, but the prime consideration was that we both thought we might be able to influence the way a small group of students, with their whole careers ahead of them, might view disfigurement.

The Spanish artist, Alfredo Fernández, has been portraying people in a variety of unusual situations for some years. He has drawn people suffering from various forms of dementia, in order to study their reactions to their own face, and has presented his work at the International

Federation of Medical Students' Association meeting in Tokyo, at UNESCO, and at various other medical congresses.

We billed Henrietta as a consultant at Changing Faces, a charity involved in the psycho-social support of those with facial disfigurement and mentioned, as casually as we could, that she also lived with Möbius syndrome.

Once in Berlin, Henrietta and I met Alfredo for supper the night before the portraits and the next day I took Henrietta to the seminar room. It was on the top floor and looked out over a patio to views over Berlin; light would not be a problem. Around half a dozen students wandered in and sat down. I stood up to introduce the session and then we all quietened down as the portrait began. Henrietta sat as Alfredo sketched her in oil pastel on a black sheet of paper. No one knew what to expect; the students were absolutely still sitting behind Alfredo. I sat at the back, offering Henrietta what moral support I could.

Alfredo worked fast. He began with one eye, huge and luminous green. Henrietta's eyes are greeny-blue but some way short of Alfredo's colour and size. Another eye. He worked quickly and intensely, pausing every so often to consider the next move. He seemed in another place, impervious to what was going on around him. We all sat absolutely silent and still, drawn in by the intensity of Alfredo's work. After 40 minutes he smiled at Henrietta; he had finished.

We all relaxed and discussion began, after a fashion. Naturally, the students found it difficult to say what they felt and Alfredo was reticent, too. He did not want to discuss his own work and, in any case, he had been concentrating so hard on the portrait that he could make no conscious judgements. The discussion went on for some time before Alfredo turned the portrait round for Henrietta to see. Seeing her own portrait was,

'Apprehensive and daunting – having been exposed to an artist looking at you intensively for half an hour with an audience watching the emergence of the picture – I had felt completely in the dark and yet very much on view. Everyone else knew, had watched, and had seen.

'Yet I was still faced with a barrage of questions. "Had he focused on the disfigurement?" "Had it been exaggerated and exasperated, what had he seen, what hadn't he seen, was it credible, was it kind?" Furthermore, the discussion had started with me still not seeing the portrait, and now not only the portrait but my reaction to it was being analysed.

'My instant response was that he had been kind, that he had created something realistic, not too strange or too unusual. I felt totally fragile and vulnerable. "What had he painted, and how might I react?" But to me, seeing it, it was OK. The relief was huge.'

One or two of the more forthcoming students had asked about the eyes. Alfredo just said that was how he saw them at the time, and that it might be different if he did it again, in five minutes time, five hours or five years. Each moment was different and his job was to capture it as best he could. The discussion moved on to what the portrait expressed. The eyes were large and rather impassive, but around the brow and the nose and mouth Alfredo's pencils had been freer and the resultant movement gave the portrait an uncertain appearance. The general view was that she was nervous.

'Of course I was nervous; but did I, could I, show it? I don't know – Yes, the situation was quite daunting, but how could that be seen with my Möbius?'

Some students suggested she must have found it difficult in front of the audience and was bound to be anxious. Henrietta agreed.

'It was difficult, challenging, apprehensive and even perplexing. How would he see me? I believe in myself and set myself up to be fairly confident but I so want and need to show my "me" to the outside world. The sheer act of placing myself in someone's else's hands was a huge responsibility and a great risk.

'I couldn't imagine how he could portray me. I was concerned that it might be a superficial exercise, which would focus simply on my physical features without conveying any essence of my personhood – or perhaps it would be the wrong essence ...'

Alfredo was less forthcoming, viewing his role as a vessel through which a portrayal emerged, through him not from him. Henrietta continued,

'We had set out with the idea that a picture evokes different emotions. Given the premise that my face does not express feeling and emotion, would it show the simplicity of portraiture and the limitations of taking a single visible image of a person? This idea seemingly did not allow for the artist's interpretation, the moods and dynamic of the situation, the subject, the artist, the room, the audience, and the time of day.

'The discussion focused on the expression and interpretation of the face – the sessions seemed intent on interpreting the artist's interpretation as a reflection on me – despite Jonathan prompting that each individual might have an independent reaction. The discussion seemed stark and, to me, inaccurate.'

No one mentioned the Möbius syndrome, being more concerned with what the face was expressing. For Henrietta this was extraordinary.

'How could they not even mention it? Did they not see it? Were they uncomfortable? Do we not respond in such a way, or indeed what constructs the image that we make of another before us? How do we perceive another being?'

Though Henrietta never moved her face, portraits don't move either[1] so, in a way, the process may have made her lack of facial expression less remarkable. After a quiet lunch – Henrietta was tired from the morning – we began again. This time there was a full room of at least 30 students; word had got around. As before, I sat near the back, supporting Henrietta as best I could.

'I was very aware of and conscious of Jonathan's presence. It was crucial for my reassurance! The process did feel invasive of my space and me but, nonetheless, I was much more comfortable and familiar with the format second time round. I was also prepared for the potential range of forthcoming responses. Confident that he was not going to desecrate me, I was still curious about how Alfredo's second image would turn out and, at the same time, intrigued how it could be different because of the clinical definition of my face. But, by this stage, I knew it would indeed be different. I had built up a nice rapport with Alfredo and felt comfortable with him. But this did not make him a mind reader. I wondered how this reflected on how people perceived me during real life.'

Once more, Alfredo was consumed by the portrait for 30–40 minutes and everyone sat completely still, entirely focused on what was unfolding before them. Portraiture is not normally considered a dramatic art, but this was. Then, as before, Alfredo stopped, smiled, and it was finished.

The larger audience was more forthcoming and commented on the eyes and the expression, thinking Henrietta was quite relaxed. Alfredo allowed her to see it straight away. She also liked it more.

'It seemed to resemble the image of me that I had in mind. It seemed less harsh – without the sadness and the implied tragedy of the first image. I do not see that in myself, and had not liked that it could have been so interpreted. I need desperately to project myself to show the real me to the world and help the spectator form his opinion and view of me accurately, and not be based on confusion or misinterpretation.'

Then we brought the portrait from the morning out for comparison. All were agreed that the second was more relaxed, with less nervousness on the face. In the afternoon, evidently, she was more at home with the situation and Alfredo had shown this. Henrietta was puzzled,

'This begs the questions: how did he know, how could he sense that – with no words, and no gesture or expression being expressed?'

I suggested that people need to look at the face but also beyond it to decide what a person was like, since only a few facial expressions were unambiguously shown on the face. I then suggested that Henrietta, having Möbius, was actually unable to move her face at all. A photograph in the morning and in the afternoon would not have shown any difference, except for lighting, and that all the differences, in emotion and feeling could only have come from Alfredo's process of portrayal and the audience's subsequent interpretation, and that it was very difficult to know how correct these were. Henrietta agreed.

'I absolutely – hugely – endorse this. The audience could not possibly be able to see physical feeling or emotion. The portrait was open to the artist's interpretation and the audience's take on it. How could they be accurate? Inaccuracies might reflect my miscommunication and their lack of comprehension of me.
'Interestingly I didn't feel that the original premise, to discuss the relation of the face and self, and especially a face with a visible difference, was addressed. Neither debate focused on facial visible difference and the confusion and lack of understanding that can occur with stereotypical attitudes and judgements made by society.'

Someone suggested that it was obvious that Henrietta was more at ease in the second portrait and that anyone would know which was first and which second. So I arranged for some of the medical students at the desk running the conference to come up to judge. They were split equally as to which was the first and which the second. The second was less free and more composed, the first looser and more expressive. But which came first and which second was not easily seen, confirming the suspicion that the audience were projecting their feelings onto it.

London

A few months later, Alfredo was visiting London, so we arranged to meet for a third portrait, one Saturday, in the offices of Changing Faces, in University Street, halfway between University College and an upmarket strip joint. After coffee and catching up, Alfredo selected a place with natural light and settled Henrietta down. As he began, the atmosphere went from the informal to one of an intense quietness, just as it had in Berlin with an audience.

Though the portrait once more took 30 or 40 minutes it seemed far quicker, as Alfredo was completely consumed by the process of drawing. As he drew, he would pause occasionally to look before beginning another burst of activity. Henrietta sat there. What was she thinking, I asked later?

'Mostly I was in my face, trying to relate to Alfredo.'

I wondered what it was to be in the face, especially in a face which did not move, or express.

'I wanted to project me – what I am – very much, through the face. At times I am thinking at a deeper level, far away from human interaction but when I am in the face it is a physical feeling, I feel myself projecting outwards, trying to convey, to exteriorize.[2] In looking at him I am trying to show him through my eyes. I wanted him to see me.'

Alfredo, for his part, could feel the intensity of the space between them change during the drawing. Henrietta also felt this.

'But I don't know if Alfredo could read what I was showing or trying to show.'

Then, after this incredibly intense 40 minutes, she looked at the portrait for the first time and was struck by the different colours,

'The face is pinker and the hair yellowier ...'

The portrait made her look a little younger, but also more contemplative. Henrietta thought she could see that in her face, but also saw a seriousness she was also feeling at the time.

Like many artists, Alfred was reluctant to dissect what he did. But away from the students he did open up. Some artists, he said, prefer to work from a photograph but he always worked with real people.

'I take from their eyes, their face, their movements and posture, from everything they have done together, from an aura I feel, from their energy, speech, body language, from everything I can. My first decision, when painting, is about the colours the person is showing me. Do they have make-up or not, what effect is the light, artificial or natural, having? One can see a lot from the skin, since some emotions show here, whether the red of embarrassment or the grey of tiredness. Sometimes, someone will change during the half hour of the portrait. Always for me it is a new place and new decisions.

'I work with models, and some other people, who always want to show me something and to see that something in the portrait afterwards. They will hold a smile for half an hour. I have to see behind this.'

Henrietta found this difficult.

'The surface ... I don't see how you can see me if only looking at this. How can you look at just the surface and see what I am?'

Alfredo replied.

'Normally I see a person just before I draw. I try to hold back any mental picture of who they are and not form an impression. I don't want to analyse. I just want to absorb everything and see the detail. I try not to jump to conclusions or interpret – I just put down what is visible. Everyone makes so many judgements and opinions about all the people they meet, and from these very initial observations we make conclusions and snap judgements. I try not to do this.

'When I start I do not know what will happen. They want to show me a picture – I don't know what I will see. I try not to form conclusions, but just receive. I only interpret after, when finished, my opinion is only formed afterwards.'

Alfredo was concerned that Henrietta had not given an opinion of the portrait. She struggled a bit so I helped her out. Sitting behind Alfredo, the painting had begun slowly and carefully, with one big eye then another, like a Cheshire cat, disembodied on the paper. Then, as he worked, I felt the portrait getting bigger and bigger, and more and more powerful. At one stage it seemed too big for the paper and that he was struggling to fit it in. The portrait seemed to show power and contemplation, but also a self-reliance and an austerity, as though Henrietta knew for herself the price paid for her success in the world. All this I saw, though whether it was in me or on the paper was impossible to know.

Alfredo agreed about the size.

'Sometimes I miss a part of the face or the hair off since the paper seems too small. Sometimes it is the opposite.'

Henrietta continued,

'I could not tell, and yet wanted to know, which bit he was painting, so I could concentrate on projecting myself in that. If I had known I would focus only on the nose. I look in the mirror and see my face. But I never think of the face when in conversation with others. I got no clues from Alfredo's face during the painting. No feedback.'

I wondered if there was anything passing between them, as during a conversation. I drew a diagram with lines between people. In conversation, words, intonations, gesture, and facial expression all bounce between people back and forth. In the portrait, the flow seemed very different, from Henrietta through Alfredo onto the paper in one direction only. Alfredo agreed, 'I try to put down what is felt in what is seen.' Henrietta received nothing back.

She agreed that the portrait showed an inner strength and a resolution, but was less aware of austerity. Perhaps this was like courage, a tag others gave you.

Alfredo interrupted,

'Henrietta wants actively to influence how people interpret her – but we all do.'

She replied,

'But with me there is a bigger risk that they may see something else if they only look. I don't want them to get me wrong. You talked in Berlin of other ways of communication, speech, music, gesture … But you deny me these in the picture.'

She came back to today's portrait.

'It looks more like me than the others, especially in detail and over the left side of the face. That is calmer; the right side is more complicated. I am more thoughtful in it; that is seen in the drawing. All my emotions are present.

'What did I feel when in the face? It was a physicality and something right up to and in the skin. When smiling I feel a warmth and when sad, no warmth. Seriousness is a determination and a concentration in, and on, the face. Last time it mattered to me, this time it does not, it is more an academic curiosity.

'When I want to show something, do I actually do it? When I don't want to show anything, what do I show? I was certainly showing concentration, as best I could. Did Alfredo feel it though?'

He replied,

'I paint with feeling, which others may see. I don't know what I feel as I do it … It is almost as if I have an absence of self during the process … I only see after.'

We then looked at all three portraits together. The first seemed uncertain, but more expressive, the second flatter and less intense.

Perhaps the third was the more expressive and more like Henrietta, and – maybe – showed something passing between sitter and painter. I wondered what 'being in the face' was for Henrietta.

> 'It means controlling what you reveal. Sometimes I am trying to show, sometimes not. I use my head and face in a different way to others. What do I show? You do not usually give conscious attention to the use of the face except, say, during a photograph. I am the same. But then if you are stared at for an half an hour … The definition of paralysis is no movement but to express you need to move. To express, do you not need movement?'

Alfredo suggested that,

> 'It is not necessarily more complicated in Henrietta, since others want to project something and so don't let me in or past this. The crux is the degree of liberty, of ease. How much the model is free in life to accept that you are different things, good and bad?'

I suggested Wittgenstein's statement that the most difficult thing was to look without prejudice. Alfredo agreed,

> 'We are not free enough, often enough, in our thoughts. What you want to see and what we are able to see, we are not always able to distinguish them. Thinking of beauty, we don't always see what is there, and are not always able to differentiate between what we think is there and what we want to see, and what we actually see. I try not to.'

I asked if he had been more puzzled drawing or interpreting Henrietta than with other people. Alfredo agreed, in being able to see what is to be seen, but also in feeling whilst painting and in his interpretation. He wanted to look and draw without preconceptions, without – almost – himself being there.

> 'I look inside. They may try to show me one thing but I see another.'

Knowing that he had painted a series of people with dementia I asked what he saw inside there. If he truly did look beyond, then what was there?

> 'I saw confusion, what is next, who I am, where will I go?'

I persisted; what if the dementia was so severe there was no one there?

> 'Even when severe there is something … it is terrifying to interpret no feeling, and this could be scariest for you.'

I wondered if this process was an empathetic one, trying to enter the feelings of the sitter?

> 'To an extent, but it is not the main feeling. If I see too much pain or suffering or illness I have to draw back. I understand, but not at the time. I understand, but not consciously. You can hurt someone if you see a thing and they mean another. People see different things.'

Henrietta had been surprised and slightly shocked by the process. She had always thought, and been told, that she could not express anything on her face, let alone subtle emotions. Yet in Berlin the audience had agreed on the expression and emotions in Alfredo's two portraits. Either the audience had projected these feelings onto the painting, or Alfredo had successfully introduced them, somehow, into his portrait. Either way, Henrietta had much to think about. Perhaps people are so used to interpreting facial expression that they create expressions on faces even when they are not there, just like they see a man in the moon.

> 'For a person with Möbius, where the potential for miscomprehension or labelling is high, the necessity to convey oneself accurately is enormous. It is scary for me to be so open to interpretation [from my face] with so much scope for wrong analysis.'

We had anticipated that, by showing Henrietta's immobile face, we could stress how important it was to go beyond the face to build up a picture of another and so to subvert the genre of portraiture and of image. Instead, we had been amazed at the agreement within the audience about the first two portraits. Alfredo and the audiences seemed to have found meaning on the face where none was present, seamlessly taking from the context and situation feelings that were then projected onto the face. Even when we pointed out that she could not show emotion on the face, it seemed to make little difference to them. Henrietta found this very difficult.

> 'I cannot put my best face on. I have no control. Someone else may put on that most beautiful or sexy face. I cannot do this. In communication I can control a conversation, but I cannot control anything in the portrait or through my face. It is all up to Alfredo. Were these differences there at the time of painting or did they come later? I seemed to be left with the unanswered question; was this emotion really there, did it really exist? It is so important for me that people understand me and don't form a false impression.'

Alfredo listened and then just said,

'As a spectator, what is most difficult for her to express is her consciousness.'[3]

Henrietta went away trying to work out how she could control inter-actions with others through her face, as well as through gesture and speech, to avoid others misinterpreting what they saw. After a lifetime of thinking that people took nothing from her face, and all from her intonation and gesture, she had much to reconsider. As Merleau-Ponty [1962] wrote,

We are always in being, just as a face, even in repose, even in death, is always doomed to express something.[p 452]

But 'doomed' is perhaps too gloomy; the interpretation by others of Möbius facial expression can work both ways. One woman with Möbius took her wedding photos into her colleagues at work. Someone said, 'But you are not smiling!' She had to say that she never smiled. Her colleagues had not realized this before because in a sense she did smile, not with her face but through gestures and voice.

Chapter 10

Changing of the rules

One of the experiences of some of those with Möbius, both children like Celia and Duncan, and adults like James and Clare, is a reduced awareness and experience of emotion. We now turn to three people who as adults are able to relive their memories as they developed an emotional life. Though we are now going back to consider early lives, this allows a way of understanding how these three moved from being emotionally impoverished to where they are now, richly emotional and enjoying life to the full.

Unlike Celia, Eleanor, in her late twenties and full of life, could remember little about her childhood. But she was more than happy to discuss her adolescence and adult life thus far. Like Celia, however, she thought her early emotional experience was dulled, and then triggered and developed through music.

In the fingers

'Sometimes, if you are in one state of mind, you need others to know. Emotion came for me when I played the piano. We always had a piano and I had lessons from age 6. By 13, I was quite competent and I found that my fingers unleashed emotion and expression in me, even though I did not know what they were. I would play one piece again and again in various ways; happy, sad, cheeky, all jumbled up inside.

'Musical notes and pattern imposed a mood … though not always the mood I felt. I might have been in one mood, but another would come out through my fingers; there were channels of all sorts of different things inside me. There were some sounds, often chords, which gave a feeling of pathos or tragedy; some seemed to sum up my pain.'

I suggested to her that she seemed to be exploring moods through music even before she knew what these moods were. It was as though an artist might have started off with a palette with just grey and then, suddenly, red, blue, green are there to play with. As she played with them so she began to experience them too and then, by playing with the colours, she realized what they meant. Eleanor agreed.

> 'Yes, I had to learn the palette without the feeling initially and then map feeling on. I grew up with music and heard different tones, even though I was not fully aware of emotions. Since I did not have the language, or the words, for feelings, the music and my fingers would convey them. Often what was conveyed was real pain. They could really say it. At that time, everything was in the fingers. I had no body language.'

This is reminiscent of what a speech therapist working with chronic institutionalized adults once told me. Alison Muir looked after people, often with no clear diagnosis, who had recently been released from long-term care in large psychiatric hospitals. They had poor awareness of others and no social skills, having lived for years in a largely asocial society. She noticed that they often had reasonable verbal skills but poor recognition and use of facial expression. With one man, unable to know what he felt and thought, she began, very simply, by showing him facial expressions drawn in cartoon form. Then with her hands she moved his face to a smile, making him look in a mirror to see, trying to show him for the first time a relation between smiling and happiness. She gave him a set of faces with various expressions, which he called his 'maps of feelings'. Another man who had hardly spoken for years reached for his feelings through art, beginning to speak by saying, 'Monet's picture is quiet; I feel like the picture.' [Cole, 1998][1]

Eleanor would spend hours playing the piano, scarcely understanding the emotional, private world opening out under her fingers.

> 'I think my piano teacher understood me. I loved her dearly and she let me do Grade 8. Nothing was said but I think she knew. At the time I was very unhappy, and she was a safe haven, in a warm room with the sweets she gave me. As I managed to control my emotions, as best I could, I think she heard the musicality and the emotion in my playing. I think my family must have known. It was a time when I was truly, truly unhappy. I was all alone, and had no one to turn to. The amazing step on was when I realized I could transfer this to my body and then when I moved it to the voice, though I do not know how I did this. It did not just happen one morning.'

Cake and shoes

Moving to secondary school was more than usually daunting. Her parents wrote two letters; one about games and the other about her need to sit at the front. The first morning they were all sat in alphabetical order and then, once the teacher had read the note, Eleanor was moved.

'There were six of us who had been to the same school so, at the beginning, we hung around together. The first 18 months I developed my own friends, but then came the pubescent stage and girls change. It became much harder and, looking back, two or three bullied me, even one I had known from prep school, so that was dreadful.'

Increasingly, her friends no longer involved her. On one school trip they ran away from her and then in class no one talked to her. It was so confusing because the rules changed so often. One day they talked, but another they would not. For her 16th birthday, they gave her a cake, but no one would sit next to her. She found it so painful and destructive. She had one loyal friend in another class whose mother had died and that brought them together.

'They talked about me in hushed tones: day in, day out; that is exhausting and dispiriting, and no one helped. The teachers did not do anything; they must have seen what was going on. Now there are many ways to address it in terms of inclusion and diversity, etc.'

It was very difficult since Eleanor did not want to draw attention to herself. She did not know, either, what to say.[2]

'Looking back it is as though I have this outer shell, which was the body which would go through the motions; school, homework. I spent hours in my bedroom, daydreaming happy endings I believed. I played piano and read. I had not got to the stage when I understood what the emotions were saying about my state of mind. It was very crude and all in the music.'

At one stage, she was so unhappy that she plucked up the courage to talk to a teacher. But, once there, all she talked about were the big horrid orthopaedic shoes she had to wear. Eleanor realized, some time later, that she had picked the perfect teacher. She was naïve and did not realize that this teacher was a lesbian, nor mature enough to know what that meant. But she did understand that the teacher had had to face her own problems. Then things looked up; she got a proper friend.

'I went and found her. She did things her way and did not worry if she fitted in. I had had enough signals from her that I would not be rejected. She was very sporty though she also liked reading books. Our families were totally different, which was good since we could talk about them. Her father was a pilot, so they travelled a lot. We hung about together and for two years she was my friend. I had a best friend in my sixth form. She had a car and I never drove.

'I didn't tell her what I was feeling, I could not tell her, but she had a good grasp. Obviously, the syndrome did not bother her; she had this amazing sense of the body and was a very good gymnast and went on to be an international judge. So she understood my body much more than I did and she understood about trying to get me to do things … she was out to improve my quality of life. She would work out routes of where I went so I didn't get lost. I have no sense of direction and could not see where I was very well. Her simplicity and directness were ideal. She was at ease with me and my bits that did not work. When her family all went to Seattle one summer I felt a very painful sense of absence. I had not experienced a raw emotion before. I only realized that it was an emotion once she had gone and then come back.'

The hug

'I had an old family friend, Diana, who loved me as a child. I always had the adult thing with her and we would talk about how her young daughter behaved and, since I was only 14 myself, it was strange. Once I was with her during holidays and I was near the edge, being so unhappy with myself and I tried to speak with her. But, in the end, I told a cousin instead. She obviously told this friend and there was a real shift in our relationship. Diana just gave me a hug; no one had given me a hug before.

'We would spend hours talking about everything. I found a way to articulate things to her – being different, being excluded – and when she gave me a hug I was so shocked to know what physical warmth was, to be approached through the body not through the intellect. This embodied experience was extraordinary, and the next day it startled me out of my wits. There is a whole new something out there I knew nothing about. Diana knew how unhappy I was and realized how much I needed her, and she said she loved me and it was not conditional. It meant to me that there was a worth and value to my life; at that stage I could not understand why anyone might love me, since I did not even like myself.

'That moment marked the beginning of her becoming a crutch for me. I would stay with her and her family. They are all very touchy-feely; they have always loved me, for me.'

Choice

'Though my teenage years were unhappy, I realized that there was something out there better and worth carrying on for. I had long periods of time isolated, when I carried on in a dogged way. I could have had a breakdown and refused to come out of my room. But I don't know what else I could have done, so I carried on.[3] If I had had a disagreeable day at school or the health issues were bad, I would go through the issue and cope. It was later that I would be upset. It was as though the brain went through it and then the emotions caught up and said that this was really big stuff and then I would get upset.

'I did not have the words, and I did not have anything to imitate and mimic. Yet there was something in me on a primordial level expressing pain, then later – after the event – I would get down and depressed and would cry in desperation. I never really expressed it in front of others.'

In her mind, there was no doubt that she would go to university and when the time came she chose architecture. She wanted to show everyone she was normal and could have a profession. All the universities she applied to rejected her. Her academic qualifications were reasonable, so she did not know why they turned her down. Later she found out that her head's report had been unhelpful.

Though she felt badly let down, she worked out that it would be possible to reapply after her A levels rather than before, which was more usual. Knowing that her head's report would be the same, she spent three days phoning up 30–40 universities pleading her case. She worked out a spiel, saying she had some health issues but that she was prepared to work hard. In the end two accepted her and she made her choice.

'I was aware it would be hard away from home. I could picture myself going to lectures and doing the work, but I was not sure how I would make friends. I knew people went to university and had a good time, went to parties and got drunk, and I was not sure how I was going to do that. It was going to be an adventure. But I did not have a clue how I would cope.

'I remember my mother leaving me in my room on campus and there was a note that the Freshers' dinner was that night. I did not know how to go anywhere, I only knew how to go to places I knew. I did not know how to go somewhere new. My room was OK but I sat on my bed and thought what have I got into. How can I do it? What am I going to do? I kept looking out the door down the corridor but there was no one there.

'I left the room and found two girls coming downstairs. I asked them if they were going to the meal and I asked if I could go with them and they said yes. They talked non-stop to each other and I just watched and listened. I did not know what to say, I did not have the chit-chat, but they did not ignore me or tell me to go away, so I went with them. They talked to people around us. I watched what they were doing and learnt from them. I wanted to hide the Möbius so I did not mention it. I wanted to be normal.

'After the meal the girls said, "Let's go out for a drink," and I thought, "Crikey." I had only been out with my brothers. "Let's go back and get changed," and I thought, "What do I do now? Do I put make-up on?"

I went back to the room and changed. I knew I had to go. It was all part of learning, but I did not have the guide book.

'We went to the students' bar and it was full, with loads of people all talking, and I still did not know what to do. I talked about school but I didn't have exciting stories. So for the first year I fell in with a kind of group, though they were not really my sort. But it allowed me a vacuum to watch and see what worked. Early on, I worked out that even though I did not know what to say, if I asked the right questions they would chatter and this created a dialogue.

'There was no feeling that people talked to me because they had to. There was no animosity; it was very different to school – I did not feel judged. We had all had different experiences and were from different places and different backgrounds. As the year went on, I developed tools to be more available, sometimes crude and rough and ready, but by watching I saw how people did it.

'Some people were lovely to me. I had not had people like that before. They wanted to spend time with me, they would seek me out. They would want to go shopping with me, go out in the evening with me, sit next to me. No one had ever wanted to do that before.

'I signed up at Freshers' week to all the societies. One was for computer science and a friend and I used to sit at the back and talk and giggle because the lecture was so boring. I know that is what schoolchildren do, but I had never giggled like this before. Suddenly I knew lots of people and they didn't ask me about my face. I had things to talk about since we shared a life at university. I learnt about what they talked about and did the same. There were some things I could not talk about, boyfriends, since I did not know that, but there was enough.

'We lived on campus and went out on campus, so there was a network of people who all knew each other. This was extraordinary. My image of university had been about studying and getting a degree, and yet I learnt in the first year to mix with people. I learnt about different and new experiences, interests, and cultures. I heard of abortions, single-parent families, and of poorer families. I just started talking to people. Men were more difficult but it was not an issue.

'For the first time I had the choice of friends.[4] I would go to a group, look around, and talk to someone with the same interests and you'd have common experience and could start to talk. For the first time, my identity was not Möbius, though I did not know what it was – that had not yet become defined. For a long time all my efforts had been to get to university. I had not thought how I would be once there.'

A god

'That first night going out for a drink, I did not really have anything to wear, but it didn't matter. Over the months I bought clothes like everyone else to wear, hippie clothes, and I started to develop a character. It was maybe artificial, but I could design my own. Most people's evolve as they grow up; mine I picked.

'I wanted to be someone who people would like. Before people had not liked me, so I wanted to be sweet, gentle, and likeable. I did not want to be radical – at the time there were lots like that. I did not want to stand out. I just wanted to be inoffensive, reliable, and so that is what I became. That sort of person meant that I did attract people towards me. By the time I left university I was renowned for knowing everyone and everyone knowing me. How did I go from that first night, not knowing how to interact, to that?

'I learnt body language, interaction, to be comfortable with myself. I think I developed a broad circle of friends, because I found I could express different things with different people. I did not find a single, really intimate friend to whom I could tell everything but my series of friends fulfilled different needs. Some I could talk about Möbius with, but then I also had a good friend who has no emotional intelligence and I never went there with her. By the end of my first year I met a great gang who were older than me, about to start their final year and I shared a flat with them on campus and I was part of a community and we were just normal. My face just did not seem to be an issue. This time allowed me to dissociate me from the Möbius, an interlude when I could work out how to be.'

There were disabled people around; one had fallen from a horse and lived in a wheelchair with personal assistants. Eleanor did not befriend her and had never labelled herself as being 'disabled'. She just wanted to be normal. Around this time, a friend encouraged her to apply for a job behind a university bar. She got it and will be forever grateful.

'It was the coolest thing. If you could get a drink quicker than anyone else you were a god. All the cool people worked behind the bar. I was accepted and part of that crowd. We would have our break after we had finished the bar before tidying up. It was no longer me on the edge not knowing how to get in, nor what to say. I'd be in the middle giggling and being teased and being normal. One tall, tall guy who was gorgeous, and who all the girls adored and who was a total rogue, was so sweet to me. He would pick me up and throw me around and hug me. It was a total flip from my previous life.'

To change the world

The Möbius did not completely leave; in fact at one stage she became totally obsessed with it. She began to realize that there were two parts; her visible difference and her lack of functioning as a person. She anguished over whether her lack of body language was due directly to the lack of movement of her face and whether both were part and parcel of her 'not developing'. As she learnt to become more of a person, it brought her back to Möbius.

'The past had not been nice and people's behaviour had not been right. I needed to understand Möbius. In those days one could not go to the Internet and type in "Möbius". I started to question doctors in a way I had never done before. I wanted to know about other people with Möbius. I knew that there were others, but my world had never gone beyond myself. Now I wanted to know what it meant. My world had broadened so much … I did not want to meet others with Möbius, but wanted to know more. Why had it happened, what did it involve?

'I would talk to my girlfriends and they said different things. Some would say my face was no different to theirs, but I could not buy that. Were they trying to make me feel it did not matter, or did they not see, or was it not an issue? Perhaps it did not really matter, they seemed to be saying. Others were more honest, suggesting the face was different but that it did not make me less of a person. That line helped me, since I did have a lot of things going for me. But I still had this face which was different.

'I know it sounds barmy, but I still had not realized that it was the face that was not working. I knew it looked different; I knew it was paralysed and did not do what others did, but I still did not realize that facial expression was what the face was supposed to do and what facial expressions did.'

Normally you see others' faces moving but one rarely sees one's own face moving spontaneously as it does in everyday situations. So perhaps her lack of awareness of this may be less surprising, especially since she had known no different.

'I had never looked at my own face. I needed to talk and wanted everyone to know what I had been going through. What came out was the grieving and the pain and the ostracism. One doctor gave me some articles. I did not like them, with their pictures of Möbians and of a very severe-looking Professor Möbius. He was a psychiatrist in Germany who saw the margin of society. If you looked different you were sent to him.'

She did learn from the papers, however, that something was known about the condition and that helped for the time being. She had not known, for instance, that 10% have learning difficulties. She calmed down a bit and carried on being a student. At this time, and since, Diane Breton's poem was a great comfort.

'In Search of … Face Value'

I don't get to hide behind my smile, it's invisible.
What God left out in facial expression, he added in heart.
Remember appearances may deceive.
Please excuse my face, I had to borrow it for the occasion – life.

If you're not smiling with me, you should be,
I need all the smiles I can get.
I would if I could but I can't.
You'll have to smile for both of us.

I may not know why I was made this way, but it could have been worse.
Please don't take my smile at face value.
If you think I can't smile, you don't know me well enough.

Being different may be my only saving grace.
So what if I can't smile, you can't not smile like me either!
Being able to smile would sure make things easier,
(but not necessarily better.)

If you can't see what I mean in my face,
listening is the next best thing.
You may have to listen more closely,
my face does not tell the whole story.

Please forgive me for not smiling.
I'm smiling, why aren't you?
Being me, means accepting all of me.
Vive la difference!

Smiling is a state of mind.
To those who don't know me –
my face may be a mask;
To those who do –
it may be a small impediment in communication;
To those who know me best –
it's my most unique feature.
Believe me, I'm smiling.
I am smiling, you're not looking hard enough.

c 1985 Diane Williams Breton. Reproduced with permission.
Also published in [Goldblatt and Williams, 1986].

'Then one summer I was temping for a hospital as a secretary. One day I ended up using a different terminal in an unfamiliar part of the hospital. Lots of patients came in looking for a doctor. I asked them to sit down. After half an hour, I had a room full of people and a doctor came charging in. He had been told the wrong place to go to. After his clinic, we were chatting and I could see he was looking at me. So I raised it to him, as I had never done before in front of a complete stranger. I said I have Möbius and he said he knew about it.

'It was amazing to have a doctor who knew something about it. He was charming and invited me to his home and drew pictures of the brain and explained all about Möbius. It was completely liberating for me. I just felt that there was someone who understood and who really knew what I was talking about. He was talking to me as a person and a grown-up rather than as a patient.

'Once I had this information I wanted to change the world. I wanted everyone to know about Möbius and to be treated in a different way. He said I should not do it yet, but make my life first. I learnt that I was a person from him, or at least he confirmed it. I learnt that other people had lived with the same treatment from others to me, and that there were others who had lived inside their body and their faces as I had. He was a supporter, an advocate. Sometimes you need someone to let you know you are on the right track.

'He drew pictures of what was not working and showed me that it was the face and facial expression. I realized it was not simply that the face was a different shape or form. It was what it was not doing. The things that had been focused on as a child, the eating and the speech, had been sort of perched there without focusing on the face and its expression as a whole.'

It was liberating finally to understand what the face did, but she was sad too to realize what she could not do.

'I wanted to have an operation, I wanted a smile. Dr Zucker had started doing his surgery and I had read in the papers about kids in the States having this fabulous operation, and I thought that if I can have it, then all would be OK. I wanted it even though my friends said they knew when I was smiling. I could not see this, since I did not term it smiling and I did not imagine how anyone might know that I was doing. I had no idea that people give off non-verbal signals. I had known that I needed to express, but I was not aware that I was.'

In the end she decided it was too late for the surgery, which was an important recognition that she could be herself as she was.

The years flew by, full of work and social life. At her graduation, she was with all her friends, warm and happy, feeling so good that all the hard work had been worth it and there she was with a degree, just like all the others. She would not have been human, though, if she had not thought a little of the head who had given her such a poor reference.

Chapter 11

Every second of the day

False start

In the mid 1990s, I had gone to a meeting of the UK Moebius Support Group knowing little about the syndrome. I had already interviewed a couple of people whose experiences had not been great, so I was prepared for a difficult weekend. Then at coffee I met Cate, in her thirties,[1] and as bright, beautiful, and relaxed a person as I could ever hope to meet. I talked with her and her Möbius and, as I did, relaxed. She seemed, I thought, to have cracked it.

It was her first meeting at the group and she was due to talk after lunch. She had come with her orthodontist, Jean, whom she had known since she was 2 and was now a friend. Jean had asked Cate to come to help others by her example. Cate is a singer and it was suggested she might sing a short piece; that would surely show the others what was possible. Cate was less keen.

When her time came Cate talked a little about herself to the group of around 20 or 30 children, parents, and adults with Möbius. When she had finished she was manoeuvred into singing and as she sang we were no longer in a rather stilted meeting of people with a rare medical condition, but in the presence of an extraordinary talent, of a voice full of power and beauty. Who knows what effect it had on the children present, but the parents must have seen what was possible with Möbius.

A few days later Cate wrote to me. For years, until I finished the book (*About Face*), I carried the letter round with me. It was so fiercely critical that it all but stopped me writing. Why should I think I could come to such a meeting just to gawp, to see others as interesting medical specimens? How dare I? Why should I have asked her some questions about Möbius, some of which were probing? It went on in similar vein, wounding as it went.

I am always aware that to portray people with unusual conditions one must be sensitive to their needs and wants. My solution is to allow each person control over what is written and to allow them to portray themselves with as much depth and detail as they want. I always show each person all parts of what I write about them for their agreement. Cate made me look at this anew, and question my motives again and again. In the end others did want me to write their story and I finished the book.[2]

But I was still worried that I had so relaxed with her that I had misjudged her. Why had I thought that she had come to terms with Möbius; how had I got her so wrong?

Some years later, Cate and I met up again. I still felt bad that I had so misread her, though it turned out that her friend, who had known her since she was 2, had also made this mistake. But Cate was very keen to take matters further, explaining that it had been a very bad time for her before. We met several times over the years informally before she agreed to share something of her life.

A Royal Lodge

She was born in the 1960s, premature and not expected to live. When she survived her mother was told to put her in a home and forget about her. Of course, she didn't listen and, when Cate was 8 months old, found a sympathetic local GP who referred her to Great Ormond Street Hospital (GOS) where a neurologist told her mother that Cate was as bright as a button. From there started regular visits to GOS.

She needed eye operations to correct squints, blocked tear ducts and to protect the eyes, since her lids did not close. Having a rare condition, she was asked on frequent occasions if she minded junior doctors looking at her. She and her mother never refused, though Cate was, at times, furious with the way it was done.

> 'Many neurologists were so patronising. I felt so undermined. I was wheeled out as a child on numerous occasions to be prodded and poked. In front of others, horrendous, I hated it; they don't talk to you but about you and they treated me as if I was an idiot. One doctor asked me if I knew what was wrong with me. I clammed up, how could I know at 8? I tried not to be shown at meetings as I got older.'[3]

Her father worked for the Queen Mother as a steward and they lived at Royal Lodge in Windsor Great Park,

'It was a gorgeous place to grow up. We had Police protection on the gates. There were six houses and then half a mile away was the Queen Mother's house. We had access to the swimming pool when she was not there. Whatever happened at school we had a free rein at home. There were only five children living at Royal Lodge, so we had to play with each other. People did not ignore you.'

Few people had cars, so they were almost cut off. Two buses a week, on Tuesday and Saturday, took them into Windsor, so there was not much to do, except climb trees. Cate's coordination was poor and at 11 she fell 40 feet trying to cross a narrow ledge and ended up with a compound fracture of the leg.

She went to mainstream school, which she enjoyed for the studying, but not for the bullying.

'They used to call me Cornelius, from *Planet of the Apes*, or Wolfgang, and I'd say "Wolfgang Amadeus Mozart, thank you very much." I would never show them what their name calling really meant to me.'

Two things have lived with her from that time. When at primary school, she was wearing a summer dress and someone spat at her, thick green spume he had obviously been working on. She remembers thinking that he must think her completely worthless, the lowest of the low. Later,

'I used to take my brother to senior school; he is a little younger than me. We had a tomboyish relationship. I quite liked him even though he was my little brother, though I had no idea how he felt about me. One day he called out my name in the playground and I turned round to see him and three others standing there, and they all just stood and laughed at me.

'I prefer being called names than being laughed at. The laughing and spitting has done far more damage to me than the names. I have never discussed why my brother did that. I did not show them I was in pain. Looking back on my childhood I was often very withdrawn and shy. With friends, I was OK. When I was in front of people and nervous I would feel faint.'

I mentioned Buster Keaton and the cost of his famous deadpan face. When he was a young boy he was part of his father's music hall act. Buster would be thrown around and the joke depended on him never showing how hurt he was.

'I was not showing what I felt, and I often found it difficult to express it. As a child I did not really express emotion at all.'

She was sometimes taken advantage of. 'At junior school I had been dared once to go to the head's door and take all my clothes off. When he came out, I said I had an itch.'[4] Her response to the bullying was 'attitude'. At 11, she would throw desks at people. She was never sure if she was bullied because of her red hair, her glasses, or because she was a 'mouthy little whatnot', or because of the Möbius.

Then she discovered she could sing. At 13, she entered and won a local Arts Festival competition. Her mother arranged an audition with the Head of Singing at the Royal Academy of Music. She was so impressed that she arranged lessons for her with a lay clerk at St George's, Windsor. Cate loved singing and immediately felt that this, in some way, was her destiny.

At senior school, her music teacher was fine until Cate started formal singing lessons, when she started to give her a hard time. Cate still does not know why. Fortunately, shortly after this, the school amalgamated with a boys' school, and she had a new music teacher. The new school was good for her music, but worse for the bullying. As a red-haired, mouthy girl with a facial difference, she was bullied; being a singer just gave them another reason, and though being bullied by girls was bad, being picked on by boys was a real nightmare.

She kept going and by 15 or 16 her music teacher began to give her work as a soloist. She began to think seriously of a career in music and asked to do A-level music. He refused. He just did not think she could make it as a singer, though she might 'work in the local music shop'. Cate sat in his office having hysterics, and eventually he gave in.

'Saying no just motivated me out of sheer bloody-mindedness. Between the ages of 16 and 20 I did loads of solo work, *Messiah*, *Elijah*, the Bach *Magnificat*, with my music teacher's choral society, and at school, and I also received work from other local groups, and then within my own church choir.'

Cate auditioned for the Royal College but was turned down. She did the rounds of other colleges and tried the Royal Northern College of Music. At the end of a long day, and after several auditions, they turned her down saying that the only reason they had let her through all the rounds of the audition was that she had come a long way. 'Hmm,' she thought, 'I could have seen Manchester instead of singing and playing in front of this stuffy bunch.' The next year, after all these rejections, she was accepted by the Royal Academy of Music. 'Everyone was really surprised. No one in my family had been to university, no one from the school had gone to Music College and I got into the top one.'

In the year between school and the Academy she found a job working in a draughtsmen's office. She was the only woman and though 19, was still naïve. She found the chat and innuendo difficult, and at times all but impossible.

'I'd often wear very frilly feminine clothes, and my work colleagues were all 50 plus. They loved me dressing up all "girlie girlie". They also enjoyed teasing me, knowing full well that I didn't understand what they were talking about. During a coffee break, one chap said that he'd like to "break me in", and because I was so naïve, I asked him what he meant. The whole table just fell about laughing. When someone at the table did explain, I was so embarrassed.

'I did, however, become very friendly with one guy. We had lunch together every day, and he was kind and gentle, and made a gorgeous apple strudel, which he used to bring in. I kept in touch with him even after I had left. I really just saw him as being a friend – after all, there was a 34-year age gap. During my first term, I invited him to my digs and I greeted him with a kiss on the lips. He leapt on me.

'I was so shocked that he found me attractive, and that he did not want to have a cup of tea first. But I managed to stop anything untoward happening and we had something to eat, and then we went to the Academy and then he tried it again, so I sent him packing. For me, the big thing was about kissing and taking my glasses off. Sex was a big issue too, but it was the kissing and the face that really frightened me.'

Unwanted and unexpected advances aside, she found the whole 'men at work' thing difficult, but survived, partly, by thinking of her place at the Academy. Starting there, however, was a shock.

The Royal Academy

Living in a hostel with 60 others, with the constant noise of practice and an atmosphere of young egos competing, was more pressured than she had anticipated. She found it intimidating to listen to others the whole time, and she began to feel enormously insecure. Her main problem, though, was not at the hostel but at the Academy.

'A singing lesson is so very intimate, between two people, and it is all about the mouth and how you stand and so is very visual.'

Her first teacher never made an issue of the fact that Cate, without movement of the lips and with half her tongue paralysed, had to use her vocal apparatus differently.

'My first year was fine; Edith would start and end each lesson with a big hug. She would say things like, 'Sing Albert Hall,' which meant that I had to project the sound. Her eccentricity made me laugh. She was lovely, but at 72 she couldn't demonstrate anything, and together with her equally old accompanist, it made for almost riotous lessons. I did not feel too scrutinized; it was all so funny.

'At other times I had to sing in front of others, during repertoire classes, and was pulled apart in front of everyone on my singing, standing, look, pronunciation, etc. It was horrendous. I know this was the same for every-one, but I found this aspect of performing very hard to deal with. I bottled things up and wore wild earrings as a way of rebelling. I had a great circle of friends but I'm sure I drove them mad with my pranks.'

She survived, in part by being a joker. 'One of my favourites was to wait until we were on the London underground, or in an equally public place, and let out a really loud and high note, then I would wait for people to turn round, and then I would stand there all innocent. It was such a giggle!'

At the start of her second year, she was given a very different teacher. She was foreign, so there was a language problem, and she made Cate do all her singing in front of a mirror. She had gone through her life without looking at her face, had never worn make-up and did her hair as quickly as possible. She never usually looked at herself.

'I thought I looked really horrible. My face was so ugly and revolting that I never looked at it. When I went for lessons with Helga, there was a huge full-length mirror that I had to stand in front of. She made a big thing about shaping the mouth. I said that I could not do it; she would just tut, tut at me and look irritated.'

After 18 months of Helga she could take no more, feeling she was being destroyed. Every time she tried to talk to Helga, she would say that Cate did not know what it was like to suffer – she was a German Jew. Finally Cate walked out. She was given two new teachers. They had very different technical styles and suggested very different repertoire, so she was pulled two ways. One thought Cate was singing so well that she must be in love. The other was an alcoholic and had her gin and tonic on the piano each lesson, and could not remember from one week to the next what they had been doing.

Throughout this period, she had a brilliant voice coach, who said that the Möbius made no difference to her. She kept Cate together and helped her approach a song properly.

> 'It's not just simply the case of learning the notes and words; you really have to get deep inside the music, and get to the heart and soul of the piece. You really have to put yourself in the composer's shoes, and ask yourself what he really wants [you] to do with this particular phrase. Approaching pieces in different ways was really exciting, getting to the nitty-gritty of a piece, and really understanding the style of a particular composer. The music was often passionate, and I suppose it was during these sessions that I started to experiment a bit with emotions.
>
> 'Until this point, although the sound that I was producing was reasonable, there wasn't any light and shade, and if I was asked to put more colour into my voice, most of the time I didn't know what was required of me. I think it was a question of Tina putting ideas into my head, and then I would try them out with my voice, and then if the sound I made was right, she would ask me what it felt like. I felt like I was being led somewhere I had never been before, and she was so incredibly patient with me if I didn't understand.'

These lessons were balm compared with her formal teachers. She entered her third and final year to more problems. 'The place was full of prima donnas, they would all be walking round practising, saying, "Look at me", even in the canteen.'

She also found the emphasis on her look rather than her voice increasingly oppressive. The dress code for instrumentalists was relaxed, but the singers had to dress in a certain way, with women in skirts. They were also advised about hairstyle and told that they could not wear glasses for concerts. 'It was horrendous. I was so traumatized that I only did one concert while I was there. It was always about my face.'

Despite all this, she asked to stay on for a fourth year, wanting to show she could do it. The vice principal said that he really admired her, but because of her face there were some areas in music that she would not be able to do. He said that they discussed this at her original audition.

> 'I cannot begin to describe how angry I was. If they had said no from the beginning it might have been easier. At that stage, I hadn't told a single one of my friends about my condition, so I just had no one to talk to. I walked out of the office, and went into a practice room on my own and

EVERY SECOND OF THE DAY

just sat down and cried. I couldn't even speak about this to my family. I felt totally desperate and alone.'

She had fulfilled all their expectations in singing, but they were turning her down because of her face. What was worse was that there was a deaf but pretty instrumentalist in the year above and Cate saw all the praise heaped on her. Being deaf, she thought, was less of a disadvantage for a musician than looking different. She kept going back, pleading with them for a fourth year.

'I had already been given solo work. I could do it; I had been paid for it. Why were they saying I could not do it when I had done it for four years before? I did not want to do opera anyway. The irony of it all was that four days after I had originally made my request, I had to pull myself together, and do a John Ireland prize. I came fourth, and even with this affirmation of my ability as a singer, it didn't help my cause.'

She already played piano and took up the cello and then the organ, showing them her determination and bloody-mindedness. But with poor coordination and a big problem looking up at the music while trying to look down at her fingers, let alone trying to move her feet to control the organ pedals, the latter was not a success. When she followed the notes across the page she had to move her head back and forth and got motion sickness. After a few lessons, her lovely old organ professor suggested that they use the lessons for her to sing while he accompanied her on the organ.

'In front of God'

She left and found a job in the music hire library. She worked with composers and was often the first to touch a new manuscript, which was so exciting. In this music world there was no stigma about appearance. Her boss was wonderful – and the campest man she had ever met.

'He was so wonderful and supportive. We became very close, and I went round on numerous occasions to his house for dinner parties, which were always great fun. One night we stayed up all night just for the sheer hell of it.'

After a year, Cate found a teacher who taught at Trinity College of Music. Then, after a couple of years, he suggested that Cate try for Trinity. Four years after leaving the Royal Academy she auditioned and was given a place. She also had a scholarship from the Countess of Munster, for which she was interviewed by Janet Baker.

'I was the only singer to get one. I was in awe at having to sing in front of her, since she was my heroine. I cracked on all the high notes and she asked if I had a problem with my head register. I just said how nervous I was. It was like singing in front of God. She ignored Möbius totally and did not mention it.'

That year she also joined a chamber choir called Voices Theatre Company and performed regularly with them. She soon became their main soprano soloist, joined the committee, and managed their publicity. Being a full-time student and working for the company in the evenings and weekends was more than enough.

Though smaller than the Academy, Trinity had the same pressures in performance and the same focus on looks, and provoked the same feelings. After one year she left, in severe debt, and for the next three years she did telephone sales, selling advertising space for charity. It was commission based, so no sales meant no money. Her boss offered cocaine to the staff. When Cate confronted him in his office he got out a knuckle duster and told her that no one would hear of this or else. Soon after, one lunchtime, she left without telling him. Unfortunately, she had the office keys with her. He phoned and threatened to break down her door if she did not return them.

She was so broke she couldn't afford singing lessons. She wasn't getting singing work despite auditioning, either, so she would hire a church venue, put a programme together with her accompanist, do the publicity, and then put on a recital. Nothing and no one would stop her singing.

Wrath

I asked what it was that was so wonderful about singing. She took a deep breath.

'It makes me feel alive. It is so physical. Normally my left side is weak and I feel tired. But when I'm singing I feel as strong as a carthorse, I am a six foot stunning blonde; when I'm not singing, I am five foot nothing and me. The diaphragm is such a huge muscle I feel so much power. When I sing I get this absolutely gorgeous tingly sensation all over, it is wicked. It's a lovely feeling.

'When I am talking I am very conscious of having to make the face work, because of the problems moving the tongue and lips and in making the sounds to allow others to understand. When I am singing I don't notice this. I am flying. I am away.'

None of this, yet, actually involved the sound she made but the physical, embodied act. She went on.

'I love the sound I produce now, however that hasn't always been the case. The voice can reflect any tension within the body, and certainly up until a few years ago, I was carrying a huge amount of tension. My voice didn't feel as free as it does these days, and it was so unreliable to work with as an instrument. I adore listening to music too, though the feeling is less. Often, when I'm listening to a piece of music that I have done I experience some of the feeling that I get when I'm actually performing. Very often I have to join in simply to experience the whole feeling.'

When she was singing, there was no Möbius.

'It feels as though someone else is there with me, it is very spiritual. I find it incredibly easy.'

I was interested in her singing, not technically – though her ability to sing was simply stunning – but because much of what she did was so full of emotion. How, I wondered, did she learn about emotions she may not have directly experienced?

'Singing is all about feeling. With a piano you can see the hands moving, in singing you can't see the moving parts. All the feedback is about feeling. I don't think I realized that I actually had a problem until I did a concert with five other singers from the Voices Theatre Company, in 1991. It was a semi-staged concert of opera excerpts. I was fine with my solos, and doing duets with the other soprano and the mezzo, but I had tremendous problems working with the tenor and bass. Two duets in particular, with the bass, made me cringe. They were very seductive, and I was very uncomfortable being in close proximity to a man, and to have to make love to him through the music.

'How could I do this when I didn't know what to do to attract a man, let alone seduce him? I spoke to my flatmate about how wooden and reserved my performance was. She suggested that I should turn up at the next rehearsal in something racy. I chose a cropped plunging top, and figure-hugging trousers.

'Well… when I arrived, the musical director, who was a rather large woman in her late fifties, and also the other soprano, looked at me with utter disgust, but the reaction I got from the chaps, and from Ralf, the bass, in particular, was staggering. His eyes were on organ stops. At 62, he must have thought his luck had changed. He basically couldn't keep his hands off me. So, over the coming weeks, in the safe and secure environment of rehearsals, with a professionally trained actor guiding what we were doing, and other people present at all times, I suppose I used Ralf as a way of tentatively exploring my sexuality. At the same time though, I was totally afraid of these new feelings, and spent many of the rehearsals in tears, simply because I was so overwhelmed.

'I think the way that I managed to rein back on emotions through my singing was to actually have the courage to show them in the first place. Everything was extremely raw at first, and the only emotion I initially found easy to show was pain. Whenever I was putting a recital programme together, it was always predominantly full of tear-jerkers. Not exactly a bundle of laughs for the audience to listen to, and more importantly, sometimes when I sang, it actually moved me so much that I would burst into tears.'

She worked with one pianist, Rita, for many years, from 1983 until 1997, when she moved to Germany. During a solo recital, Cate would have to sing about all sorts of feelings; she found it horrendously difficult to switch between different emotions, and relied on Rita's patience to do it at all. Even now, once she has experienced and expressed emotion more fully she can sometimes get carried away singing, and have to put the brakes on.

'I feel everything so intensely now. I used to feel that expressing emotion drew too much attention towards me, and because of Möbius I did not want to do that. Singing about love, and sexual love, was for me really alien. So I held back and was enormously frightened.'

It is difficult to imagine expressing an emotion fully in song, if it could not be experienced in oneself. 'I would agree, even though now I think I feel too much.' I mentioned that some with Möbius are unable to express emotion except as huge uncontrolled eruptions.

'I was like this. These days I find it difficult to contain emotion rather than express it. Underneath my small frame I feel like a 6'4" Russian shot-putter. I can be so high that people have sometimes said I am drunk, and when I am low it can be so dark and painful.

'I had an awful experience whilst I was studying at Trinity. During a concert, seven of us were required to do the seven deadly sins. Unfortunately, they gave me wrath to do. We basically had to recite words, and act out the sin. I had been very dramatic during rehearsals, so much so in fact that a couple of people had commented that they were convinced that I was heading towards a nervous breakdown. The performance was very much worse. With adrenalin pumping, I went for it like an absolute maniac. I picked up a large wooden chair and threw it across the stage. Luckily for me it didn't hit anyone, but the chair did break, and I screamed so loudly, I could barely speak. The musical director thought that it was absolutely marvellous, but I can tell you, I was definitely in my coach's bad books for abusing my voice. I really felt totally unable to stop, and this was very frightening indeed.'

Containing, experiencing, expressing, controlling emotions, Cate – through music – was learning not only about how to express what she was feeling, but to feel itself. And as she did this it was as though she was learning how far she could go. Since she could not express momentary elation or, say, slight disappointment, this might have led her to a reduced experience or, at least, expression of these. Perhaps she had needed music and performance to communicate and through this she learnt how to communicate in other more subtle, soft, and instantaneous ways. She agreed.

'Exactly. I find myself staring at faces now and I love it. I have to remember to blink, since I can hold my eyes open and if I am not careful I can stare for so long that my eyes start watering. There is no sadness that I cannot move my face. The only thing I feel sad about is people judging me and putting a label on me and treating me as a simpleton. In the acting profession, you can have all shapes and sizes. I thought in the music business it would be the same, but it is all about the face and what you look like and what you are wearing. It is almost obsessive…

'In my early twenties I was frantic to get work: now the pressure is not there and I don't see life the same. It is the journey, not getting there, which is important. You can miss so much on the way if you just concentrate on the finishing post.

'At the Moebius Support Group, by focusing on my face and my voice I felt they looked at me as though I was a performing pig. It was then that I started to find out more about myself. They saw a Möbius face being successful, whereas I was a successful person independent of the face.'

The letter

Before we met, she had emailed about our first meeting and her subsequent letter.

'I don't know if it's something to do with having Möbius, or whether it's just part of being me, but I have always had a bit of an issue with showing emotion, especially quite deep, painful emotion. I used to just bottle things up until everything just exploded.

'I know you will want to talk about our first meeting, and I have been going over and over in my head what happened then, and subsequently, and even after all this time, I still feel a great deal of pain about it. The worst aspect of all is what I personally did to you, and the hurt and pain that I caused you. At the time, I was hurting very badly, and I don't even think I was aware of it. You came along, and hit the right buttons, and I just went pop… Thank goodness!

'I don't think I can even put into words how grateful I am to you for what you inadvertently did that day. Consequently, I'm not sure whether I can revisit this at the moment 'face to face', which is why I'm sending you this email.

'What brought me to be at the conference in the first place? I had started to experience painful cramps in my arms and legs, and I spoke to Jean about this, to ask her whether she knew of any other Möbius cases that were experiencing similar symptoms. I think I was about 30 at the time, and apart from meeting a little 5-year-old girl with the condition when I was 28, I had not met anyone else. I didn't know anything about the support group, and I don't think I even understood what Möbius actually meant. Was I in denial at that time? Looking back, I think I definitely was. It's not that I wasn't aware of having a problem, but I saw it only on a physical level, i.e., problems with my eyes, and having muscle weakness, and not being able to move my face in the way that everyone else does.

'When I was suddenly confronted with a roomful of people with Möbius, and I listened to people such as you talking about the condition, I wanted to stick my fingers in my ears and scream out, "NO!!!!" I suppose I have always been able to hide my feelings very well, which when I look back on it now, is a very stupid thing to do. Obviously Jean, who has known me since I was 2, thought that I was "sorted", as she suggested that I go on the afternoon panel to talk about the condition, and my experiences.

'Unfortunately, she didn't ask me first, and consequently, when I arrived and saw my name down, my stress levels went through the roof. Without going into a huge long account about that day, I felt as though my whole world was crashing down. Suddenly I was being treated differently. I didn't want to be identified in that way. I saw myself purely as a classical singer, trying desperately to get myself "off the ground". I wanted to be taken seriously as an artist, and I didn't ever want to be known as the singer with Möbius.

'When I started to talk to you, and you started to ask me why I had chosen to perform, when it is such a visual profession, I initially wanted to explode. I thought, if you had heard me sing, you wouldn't even be asking me this question. You brought back that awful memory for me, when I was at the Royal Academy of Music and I asked for a post-graduate year. The vice principal told me that I wouldn't be able to have a postgraduate year, not based on my singing ability, but on the fact that they thought that there were areas in music that because of my disability, I would not be able to get into. Rather than dealing with this, I had set out to 'prove them wrong'. Not a very healthy attitude to take, and as the years were going by, I was getting more and more depressed.

'Speaking to you brought the pain rushing back. It was almost as though you had cut my head off, shaken everything about, and told me to get on with things. I had spoken about things with you that I had NEVER talked about before, and to be perfectly honest, at that particular time, I just couldn't deal with them. Music had always been my absolute rock, my safety net, and I suppose I was living a total lie. Had I fooled myself into believing I could do something... Yes I had!!! I left the conference feeling quite desperate. I dumped everything onto you, and used you as a focus of my intense pain. I know now that that was an awful thing to do, but at the time, I don't even think I saw you as an individual. I think you represented everything that had stood in my way.

'I definitely did not want to hurt you, but I did want you to feel my pain.

'It was at this point that I started to question and look at every single thing in my life. If you hadn't come along when you did, I can't honestly say what would have happened to me. I certainly don't think I would be at this stage now.

'I left the conference and got into Jean's car and tried to bottle it and got out a book and started reading, but I could not bury it. I was in a state for weeks. But I realized I had been pushing myself; not for me but just to say I can do it. If I had not met you I would have burnt myself out.'

For my part, I had been shaken by her letter, and made to examine my motives in writing about people with difference. Mostly though, I was worried that I had so mistaken Cate's mood. I thought she was so well adapted and at ease and was completely unprepared for her letter. That her friend was equally unaware, after knowing her for over 25 years, was only of limited comfort. Both of us, with varying knowledge of Möbius, had got it badly wrong.

Two boys

We returned to Cate's experience of faces now when, previously, she had avoided them.

'I love looking at faces now. I love it, it's fascinating, to watch others move. I can imagine mine moving. I imagine my eyebrows moving round, up, down at each end. When I'm talking to someone, and I see their face move, I feel as though my face moves too.'

I wondered how she did this, was it something felt or imagined?

'I am not sure, imagined. It is a visual picture, of my eyebrows, or of any-one's. I used not to look at people; I would have my head down. All my life I would hate to sit facing someone and I would never allow anyone on my left side because my left eye is not very good. I would miss out all the facial expression stuff. I would be forced to look at people during performance, but not too much.

'Now, I look at faces all the time, I love it. It's great; it used to make me feel insecure. I could not bear to buy women's magazines and see all that glam-our and beauty, whereas now I love to see the hot men on TV, and also the beautiful women. I don't see myself as I used to, some bits I like, some I don't. I used never to take off my glasses in front of people, and thought whether I would be able to do that in front of you? Now I don't mind.

'I used to worry, when I was talking to someone, about what I was looking like. But now I try to forget about me and just think about them. If I look at someone I know if they are looking at me. It makes me feel more secure; to look at someone because I know then that they are look-ing at me.'

I mentioned the same thing and almost the same words being said to me by a blind man. For him it was important that people looked at him so he had their attention. When chatting, his face was so expressive that I felt uneasy staring at him when I was unable to open myself up to him in a similar fashion.

'It happened gradually for me and a lot is down to Vin. When I went for my grant for Trinity I needed a pianist, and because I knew Vin played the piano, I asked him to accompany me. From there we started to do concerts together. I can tell you there is nothing better than playing together with someone you love. It is like having sex in public.

'He just accepted me, warts and all. We used to sit on the couch and he would start making faces by smearing his face with his hands and I would do the same. It was so funny and made me so relaxed. He showed me how to be silly with my face and not to ignore it. My face is unique.'

Cate and Vin met at Voices Theatre Company. After a while she and Vin fell out with the conductor and decided to leave to start their own choir. Starting from scratch they gave out leaflets on the streets to pub-licize it. They attracted 'all the people in the world who could not sing'. They stuck it for two years. More importantly they married a few years later and now have a beautiful, inquisitive 3-year-old boy, Ben. Cate and I were talking one Saturday morning while the boys were out bonding and shopping.

'We met on Valentine's Day 1990, and started off as friends. We were both on the committee at "Voices". We spent hours on the phone, first of all discussing choir business, and then we would go off at a tangent, and talk about everything under the sun. We'd always end up howling with laughter. Vin was seeing someone else at the time, and I was trying to pursue a relationship. I suppose gradually my feelings just sort of crept up on me. He invited me round for a meal one evening, and I went round with the sole intention of staying the night, and that's exactly what I did!

'My behaviour was very volatile when I first started going out with him. My emotions were a complete mess, and I'd either be screaming at him and walking out, or crying hysterically. I just couldn't believe that some-one would want me. He just accepted me completely, and I was able, over a long time, to accept myself completely, just as he had accepted me.

'Shortly after we got married in 1998, I started to have tests to discover the cause of my muscle cramps.[5] This was particularly difficult, because we hadn't got married until I was 35, and I wasn't sure whether or not I wanted children. As time was going by, and there still wasn't a diagnosis [for the cramps], I was beginning to think that the decision was being taken away from me. Vin was too worried about my health to allow us to start a family until we had had more information. It was a very difficult and painful time for us both. In August 2001, we asked my neurologist whether we could try for a baby. His exact words were, "Go for it girl." I got pregnant almost at once. I had a wonderful pregnancy, and our gorgeous little boy was born on Jubilee Day 2002.

'Now I don't look and see Möbius, I see I have another zit. In other words, my behaviour mirrors that of most women across the country. Last week was awful because of chocolate withdrawal. I've given it up for Lent. I look at my face now and sometimes I think I look like a bog monster, especially when I've had a sleepless night with Ben, whilst at other times I think, "Hmm, not bad!!" It is completely different. If people comment about Möbius I say when God made me the elastic broke. I say I can move my eyebrows faster than them, and I move my whole head forward and put my face right up close to them.

'A lot is down to Vin; he kept saying "You have a dear little face," and because he said it often enough, I started to believe him. I cannot say how wonderful he is. He has given me so much.

'I love my face. I don't think I really believed this until last year. I hated having my photo taken until fairly recently. I saw an advert for one of these competitions where you can win a free makeover and photo shoot. I entered, won, and went for the session last July. Vin had to look after Ben, so I had to go completely on my own.

'Right from the outset, I was completely open and relaxed about Möbius. The make-up girl was great, but it was the photographer who was totally brilliant. I knew that he would want me to smile, so I mentioned right from the outset that I couldn't, and he was an absolute star. He made me feel so relaxed, and for 30 minutes, I felt like Kate Moss, it was wonderful. Vin and Ben turned up later in the day to view the photographs, and I liked nearly all of them. Unfortunately, at £60 each, we could only afford one.'

As I was talking my nose wrinkled up and Cate stopped me and asked me to wrinkle again. 'I find it fascinating. It is so beautiful, like a piece of music. I don't wish I could do it, I just look at it and think it's lovely. Vin tells me off for staring at him.

'I cannot imagine falling in love without my face being a big part of what goes between us. Previously, I would not let anyone come close to me; I was scared of them looking; I was scared of any intimacy. I knew that men found me attractive, but I honestly couldn't understand why. When Vin and I started to see each other, the physical aspect of the relationship was absolutely terrifying. It took years before I felt comfortable about Vin looking at me and touching me. I found it so difficult to understand how he could find me attractive when I viewed myself as being so ugly.

'Thinking about it, if I had not had Möbius, I would be an extrovert. If I had not been to the Academy, I would not have been so introverted. I had spent my life denying Möbius. Now I can happily admit that I have Möbius, and I love it, I am proud of it, I am wearing a flag, and it is me. Part of me, I'm proud.

'I had spent my life in my body, in my voice, but not in my face. I had grown up with Möbius, but it was just a name. There was no Internet and I had no medical books. So I suppose I had been going through my life in ignorance, although in this case, ignorance definitely wasn't bliss.

'For me the only annoying aspect of Möbius is saying it. I always find the 'm' and 'b' really difficult to say, and nine times out of ten, I have to repeat myself. Why could it not be Jones syndrome? I just say I have some problems with my facial muscles; I don't say Möbius.'

Vin and Ben returned from the shops. After relaying the mayhem Ben had caused during the morning, Vin said,

'At choir, if she was not there and someone said a joke, and if we thought she would like it then we would imitate Cate's laugh, by leaning forward and slapping the table with a hand. She was a bit hyper when I first met her. But she has an innate quality magnified by Möbius. She feels every second of the day and has a tremendous vibrancy.'

Vin made lunch and chatted whilst Cate fed Ben, with Bach playing in the background.

'When we decided to marry in church I said we should start going regularly. The first time we went, as soon as we started singing a hymn everyone heard me. I felt embarrassed, because people would ask what I was doing musically, and I wasn't doing much, and I worried they might think me lazy. Gradually over time though, they would say I was singing to the Glory of God.'

It was a great relief to be able to think that her singing did not have to be in front of an audience. She felt that she had been given a gift.

'Who cares if I am not singing in front of huge audiences? My only regret is that I would like to do more concerts with Vin because I love performing with him.'[6]

As I left Vin mentioned, casually, that he had never noticed that Cate had no facial expression until she mentioned it.

'All of us, at times during the day, have moments when we drift or switch off, when we are doing or feeling less – dead moments.[7] I have never met anyone with fewer dead moments than Cate.'

Chapter 12

Not about anything

A foreigner

When I met Lydia, she was in her late thirties. She began talking about her life after university. She had really enjoyed Oxford and, a little like Eleanor, had created a new self, vibrant, social, and independent. She was so relaxed there that she had not thought what was next in her life. Her plan had been to go to university and prove people wrong, and she had certainly done that. It was a shock that then, in the 1990s, there was a recession. She applied to the civil service, and for jobs in publishing and the theatre in London. She sent application after application without being asked to an interview.

So she went home to live with her parents. This created rather more difficulties. She found it very difficult to be her new confident self at home when her family were unused to it. They also lived in the country and, being unable to drive, Lydia was trapped. She did some agency work as a secretary, which gave her enough money to visit friends at weekends. Mostly, during the week, she felt in a void.

Her friends suggested that she should try teaching English as a foreign language, TEFL. She was not keen, since it had a bad press at the time. But, after eight months or so, nothing was happening so she applied to do a short intensive course.

'The first interview, in Chester, I did brilliantly. There was a man who asked the questions and a silent, observant woman. They wanted to know if I could manage students from abroad and whether I could encourage and relate to them. They did not ask about the face. They did not get back to me, so after a few days I phoned them up. The lady was really embarrassed and awkward and said that I had not got the place. I knew they were desperate and on paper I was a strong candidate. I was surprised but did not pursue it.

'Five years later I was working in Spain and an examiner came from England. We were chatting on the phone and suddenly she said, "It's you,

I always thought about you and knew we had done the wrong thing."
I had no idea who she was. She said, "You came for that interview in
Chester. We had really liked you and wanted to take you. But the boss had
thought that a lot of students were from the Far East where disability might
be a problem." She said she never forgave herself, since she could see my
potential, but she did not fight my cause. Now she is my friend and mentor.'

After one interview they said she was very good, but they were not
going to take her because of her face. She had no answer.

'Now I would talk to them about the condition and what it means; how
I am as a person and how I compensate for the reactions of other people.
Instead of facial expressions I use my hands and shoulders, and my voice,
both in its tone and what I say; I construct it all very carefully. If nervous
then I sit upright on the edge of a seat. I am very aware the whole time.
I am looking at you with my eyes and making sure I am engaged with
you. My voice I use to reinforce emotion again. When I want to make a
point I really concentrate on my voice and intonation. I have to monitor
all these things constantly the whole time.

'Normally, you are responding to various signals but are not aware of
how much you are giving. If I am not getting the right messages from
you then I have to up my expressions. None of this is automatic. Because
I have to think about every sentence, and how I am to deliver it, my verbal
fluency probably slows down. I think it is tiring but it is what I have to
do. So now I can explain when I meet people that I put them at their ease
and show them who I am.'

She returned to her story.

'By now I was 23 and had started to learn to do that. At this stage it was
like learning another language, but not like my French when I had a dic-
tionary and could look up the word; here I had to invent it and work out
what worked. I had to learn register, the use of the appropriate language
and expression for the situation, whether for my father, or a friend, or
a vicar. I learnt all this. At university, people just took me as I was. Once
I had left I had to start again. At some interviews in London they just got
straight down to it; my face and I was lost.'

Eventually, she found a small language school in Pimlico. The man
who offered her a job did not mention her face at all. She still couldn't
work out why one person did one thing and another was different. But
she had a job, and made a good friend on the first day.

'I am very language-y. We started with Polish and since I knew a little
Russian that was fine. But then we had to make a presentation in front of
everyone and that was awful since everyone would look at me ... I don't
think at university I had ever been made to stand up in front of others.

This was a group of 12 to 15 who were going to look at me. I watched others go in front of me and some were quite good and some were less so. I got cross with myself because I was getting het up; it was very intimidating. But once I had done it everyone clapped, and they didn't clap anyone else. I knew then it would be OK. I did my course and passed. Since everyone was working abroad, I decided to as well. I did a summer course for teenagers and I was fine, in a role with a purpose. I loved working with students from the Mediterranean – Greece, Italy, and Spain – they were so vibrant and expressive.'

Her first post was in Greece. When she got there, the job had disappeared, only to reappear once she was home; they made up some reason. But she was not too upset, since by then she had realized how much she loved teaching Spanish students; they were always having fun with lots of parties. When she visited one student in Spain, the family made her feel so welcome that she felt none of the awkwardness she had in England. There her face was not an issue; she had found a place where she could just be herself. So, on returning to the UK, she applied for jobs teaching English in Spain and was soon offered three. She chose one in a small shipbuilding town near Santiago de Compostella. The director of studies met her for the first time at the airport and did not mention her face. Next day she started work.

'I had started to pick up Spanish quite quickly. I found it quite easy to learn languages. I used to teach in one-to-one classes and I would meet a Spanish person and we would spend an hour speaking English and an hour Spanish.'

The school had a contract at the local shipyard and she used to teach the young engineering graduates technical English.

'The first day had gone quite well. But then the manager phoned up and asked what the problem with my face was. They did not tell me, but I had already picked up that something was going on; if you have been talked about behind your back at school for years you develop radar for it. I knew my face had come up and wondered what I was going to do. They were obviously wondering whether to send me home. I thought I should bring it up, but I did not have the language – even in English – to say something I wanted to say, "Give me a chance, it will be OK."'

When they met, the managers agreed that her face had indeed been brought up but that they had decided to give her a chance. Then after a few months they renewed her contract and she spent a further two years before leaving to help set up her own school nearby.

'Now, people ask how I could work in another country. I did not think, I just did it. The big thing for me was going to university. When things are going well, you don't focus on Möbius, and in Spain they were going so well.'

But even then, she added, the problems with others and Möbius occasionally appeared, as if from nowhere. Once she was in the Canaries on holiday, walking down a street with a friend, when some woman started laughing at her and said in Spanish that people like Lydia should live in trees. Her friend did not understand but Lydia had been catapulted from enjoying a lovely holiday to feeling awful and offended.

> 'Any nice cushioned feeling had gone. The Möbius is never not there. At any time we can be getting on nicely with [our] day and you get someone looking at you in a funny way. People may not be able to understand me. It is always there. It is the amount of effort and work that I do the whole time that makes it ever go away.'

Mapping feelings

Away from home and from England, she remembers Spain as being the first time she had been completely independent. Her love and assimilation of Spanish culture allowed her to develop in ways she never knew existed.

> 'I do not think I had emotion when I was a child but now I have it. How did I get it? It was in Spain. I learnt Spanish in two months but – more – they are so theatrical in their emotional expression. The body language I had learnt and used at university could be exaggerated in Spain, using the whole body to express one's feelings. Over here in England it would be over the top, but there it was fine and because of this I learnt to feel within me.
>
> 'At Oxford I had learnt a lot of imitating and mirroring and copying but had not, to a very profound depth, had the feeling. I had been using it to conform and because if I did it I got the response, but I, myself, wasn't feeling. But in Spain everyone is so dramatic. If something awful happens then the world is coming to the end, and if fine you party all night. If sad you burst into tears and then go off to the pub. I had gathered all these skills in language and gesture and then in Spain I could just be me.
>
> 'Because of the cultural 'up-regulation' of feeling into gesture I learnt to feel. I am not sure how I mapped gesture and feeling onto my body, but I was starting to feel then. I could feel really ecstatic, happy, for the first time ever. Before, without the expression, I had found feeling difficult. Once in Spain I certainly had the means, the channel and the vehicle, and the feeling. Before, my thought was frigid or cold. I needed the continuation of a thought into real-time expression within the body.'

Darwin said that an emotional feeling can either be expressed, continued and become exaggerated or, if not expressed, reduced and lost. It is as though it has to be in the continual present, continually expressed to be continually experienced.

> 'That was how it was for me. I was an intellectual at university. In Spain I experienced emotion. As a child I used to play a musical instrument with emotional expression, but the emotion did not really come from within. I could not let it out. Now, once I could express there was no stopping me.'

Lydia's new experiences were not, of course, within her or about her alone. They emerged within a rich social, cultural world. In a place where emotions were communicated publicly more than in the UK, she learnt, somehow, to experience and as well as imitate feelings.

> 'When you live and share emotion together then you all experience it together. I met a man with Möbius who lived in Sweden and he was one of the saddest people. He was completely wooden, with no body language, like a puppet. I met him in Italy; I hope he learnt something from them. If I had not lived in Spain I don't know how I would have turned out.
>
> 'In Spain, ironically, though they use gesture a lot, they talk in a much more monosyllabic way than here. They are not as musical in speech. My voice is melodious and I had begun to use it to control people's response. So, in Spain, they all talked about my voice and loved it. That was a eureka moment. My voice could be my thing, my tool, my vehicle of expression. The voice was the link from me to other people for feeling and for emotion. The language and words don't do it. I had those in Oxford. It was the voice, the melody going with the embodied gesture, that completed the circle.'

She learnt that in her classes she could show, through her delivery, the emotion she wanted them to learn, anger, pity or whatever. She also reinforced it with flash cards. She would start off with cards of an elephant or a rainy day but then would introduce pictures of emotions, basic faces with tears, happiness or sadness. These all helped though, really, she was revealing her emotions through her voice.

Meeting Möbians

Whilst in Spain, purely by chance, she saw a TV documentary about a boy with Möbius. At the end they gave a number for any others with the condition to contact. She thought for a long time but then decided to get in touch.

'I knew the media would be interested; after all I was a young Englishwoman with Möbius, running her own business. I ticked lots of boxes. But I did it to meet someone else – for the first time at 28 – with Möbius. The TV people came and did the "English girl opens Language School" piece. It was quite fun filming, though I did not like the end result as they cut it to be sensational. I did not like seeing myself on TV either; I was made to watch my face.'

After that, 25 more families contacted them and they set up a Spanish support group. Their first meeting was in a small hillside hotel in November; they ended up being snowed in. Having been influential in organizing it, Lydia was surprised by her own feelings.

'It was tough, seeing other people with Möbius, really tricky. I did not want to be there. I loved talking to the mums and dads, sisters and brothers, and to the doctors, and they thought I was amazing, seeing what I had done with my life. But seeing others with the face was really difficult. I had not seen that before, I did not really see the Möbius in my face, but I did in others.

'I had read by then very different accounts by Möbians and had found out about the US support group. I had heard of people going to the meetings and finding someone else who had gone through the same experience wonderfully reassuring, like finding a brother. I was not looking for that. I was, by then in my late twenties, living in a foreign country, running my own business, with lots of friends in the UK and in Spain. If I was looking for something, say a partner, then that was nothing to do with Möbius. I was in a little hiatus from Möbius. I had worked out how to conduct my life and interact, and though I had not completely come to terms with having Möbius, I had found a very good way to ignore it. In Spain, it was not an issue. If it came up then I found a way of addressing it; I had become cushioned from it.'

She had become involved because she thought she could be helpful. She wanted to do what she could to prevent children going through the teenage years like her. When she went she saw what it was like and was uncomfortable.

'This was the last bit of me I had not addressed. To see lots of people with Möbius in front of me I found very upsetting. Seeing the Möbius face, seeing me in various different guises, as the little child, (though I had not been a Spanish child; Spanish children are absolutely adored by all society; that was not my overt experience), as a teenager who was still seen as a child, as a young adult; all these were very difficult. Some of the young adults had been totally smothered at home and not gone on to develop a life. Some had not had all their education. One woman had been totally looked after and had never studied or got a job. Another had wanted to get out, but the family held her back, thinking she would not cope. On the other hand, one guy was fantastic. He was at university, studying maths and science. His only Möbius feature was the face. His view was, "What is all the fuss about?" His family was very stable and they encouraged him to do anything. He was a little shy and quiet. He was not dramatic, but he was at ease with himself, though less so about Möbius and talking about it. It was to be let go of that I went to Spain.'

Going to the weekend made her realize just how much unfinished business she had. On top of that, everyone else at the congress had gone with their families; being on her own was hard. But she helped as best she could, becoming a committee member. Unexpectedly for Lydia, she was also adopted as a role model, an adult living an independent life in a different country.

Once they had set up a support group in Spain, she started looking around and found that there was already one in the UK. She had not given any consideration to this before. There was also to be an international conference in Toronto. The Spanish group decided to go and so Lydia, not long after feeling awkward meeting others in Spain, went to Toronto. The Spanish had already become like a little family and she looked after the smaller children, almost as a godmother. One child developed a complex about her mouth, so she would not have anything to do with it, even refusing to clean her teeth. Her mother found some raspberry toothpaste and Lydia went with the girl to the bathroom and cleaned her teeth after which, in the end, the girl did too. Lydia liked helping. After that the mums and dads discussed their experiences with her and asked about the various care and treatments available.

'The Spanish are great talkers and would talk all the time about how they feel. That was very different to how I had been brought up. They have the vocabulary. They articulated how scared they were, how the child that had been born was not the child they had wanted to have. When should they have an operation: as a child? When the child was older and able to choose? I lived my early years again through those Spanish Möbius children, only a life I had not lived before. As the kids asked me how to say a smile I would tell them about when I had been unable to do it. That was cleansing for me and not something I had expected at all.

'In Toronto, there were 500 families with Möbius from all over the world. It was surreal; up to the previous year I had not met a single person with it. You know what the Americans are like, "Hi, I'm Cheryl," in your face. Everyone just talked about Möbius. I was able to hide a bit since I was translating into Spanish. We got friendly with the Latin Americans. I met the group from Brazil who had done some work on the association between the drug misoprostol for abortion and Möbius.'

Apart from translating into Spanish and being a godmother, she also learnt a lot. There was an orthopaedic surgeon discussing operations for a club foot and speech therapists looking at ways to help with speech and lip closure. One man gave a talk with videos with different appliances whilst another discussed his operation. There were adult sessions too, though she avoided them with her translation work. Then she was asked onto the International Board. She sat fascinated, watching the reserved Icelandic group with the ebullient Argentineans. She had gone in a few short months from having not seen another Möbian to meeting and mixing with 500. So much happened that she hardly slept.

Piece of meat?

She returned to Spain ready to take all these new ideas to those who were unable to make the trip. She was also more confident in herself and in her life with Möbius.

'I believe passionately that it is wrong to discriminate against people because of how they look. I want to put something right. It is my moral responsibility. I discuss my experience as a teenager, when the teachers did not help. Well, they could have. I talk of the doctors who treated me as a piece of meat; that does not have to happen. No one needs to be ostracized.

'Möbius has given me a huge insight into the extremes of life. I savour and cherish the things which are most important to me. To me the face is not an issue. It is tiring that I have to make more of an effort to put my point across.

'Now, Möbius is not about anything. It is about my life, enjoying the things that make me happy, about being successful. But there is a caveat; all the physical things that go along with it, the feet, the colds and the bronchitis, like the tiredness, which is an issue. That, for me, is Möbius, not my face.

'I am as expressive as I need to be: I have lots of friends, go to the theatre, the pub, drink too much wine sometimes, go on holiday. I would like a family of my own one day.'

How to live with but not within Möbius? Lydia's answers seem as good as any.

Chapter 13

Rusty old car

It is said that for some with spinal cord injury the first 'step' in rehabilitation is to accept that you may never walk again.[1] One person with Möbius suggested that her journey to live with it began when she accepted that she was never going to be like everyone else. For years she had thought – or continued to make believe – that there was nothing wrong with her face and that others would eventually realize this. Only when she threw this away did she begin. Each person with Möbius will have made their own journey, but in coming to terms with it there are some generalizations that may be made.

It seems important to learn as much as possible about the condition and what it means for you. Remember that, even now, for some the diagnosis is only made as an adult. For children with Möbius, their parents or carers need to find out about it and communicate its effects with the child, as best they can, though how a child can understand is difficult to contemplate. One person with Möbius was told by her brothers that she could not catch a ball because she was a girl. In fact, her Möbius vision and somewhat clumsy reach made seeing and moving her arms towards a ball impossible. Just knowing what limitations Möbius imposes can allow a person to get on with their life. The more information children and their parents can assimilate the better.

More than one person has thought they were the only person in the world with this problem. 'As a child I was aware of my [unaffected] peer group; I was always comparing myself with them, wanting to be like them. Yet I could not run around or play games and I did not know why.' This need for information and for realistic goals is not only for children and their parents and family. It reaches out to a child's teachers, special education needs support, social worker, physiotherapist, and occupational therapist; whoever is involved with the child needs to understand the impact, as Gemma's story related.

As a child, much of this is physical; about the embodiment, the eyes, ears, feet, speech, etc. There are many choices to be made in terms of treatment, whether dentistry, leg corrections, splint surgery, or speech therapy. Some treatments are invasive and need careful weighing up. One person suggested that she missed a third of her education because of them. It is not all about the big things either; children with Möbius may have more severe and frequent colds and coughs. These all reduce time for learning and for socializing or just 'hanging out'.

Each person will also have different needs. There is no right way, only ways which suit individuals and their families. Eleanor only realized that her face did not move like others as a young adult. 'No one said to me that my face looked different to anyone else.' If that had been talked through earlier it might have helped her. For James it was only late in his adult life that he realized that much of his problems were secondary to his facial problem and not to his own shortcomings.

Leaving Descartes

As people grow, their perspectives may also change, whether they have Möbius or not. As a child, Celia had her body and her self and did not relate the two. In addition to her reflections on childhood I also asked her how it was now, as an adult. Did she still feel a separation between her body and herself?

> 'No; "me" is my spirit and my personality *and* my cranky old body. The latter affects me in my lifestyle, expectations, and belief structure. I cannot do some things. Me being me is everything. I have come to terms with my body though I don't necessarily like it. But what is the point of spending your life bitter and angry and recriminating? I would prefer legs that work. I would prefer to be able to walk where I wanted. I am less concerned about my face, though I would like eyes that worked and didn't lacrimate.
>
> 'When a child, you have things done to correct things, and get them as good as they can be, say, lengthening an Achilles tendon. Adulthood is about maintaining, and you have wear and tear like anyone else. But there is also more pressure, since there is less reserve and the body needs more looking after and has less capacity. Now, my Möbius body is a rusty old car that you have to keep tinkering with. Each year it has to pass its test and each time you have wobbles. I always have something going on with my body, my structure, my framework.'

If no longer a Cartesian, I wondered if she was able to assimilate her face, and yet transcend it in some way.

> 'That doesn't work for me. At the end of each day, I have to come home and look after the car again. I have to live with it. I cannot pretend that the physical constraints are unimportant. They impact on my and other people's lives. I sometimes have to say I cannot do something, say go out for a meal with friends, because of Möbius.
>
> 'It can come from nowhere – you can be going along fine and then, without warning, something appears from nowhere, e.g., the rain setting off my arthritis pain, or my balance, can lead to setback pretty quickly. It's a continual, and continuing, challenge.
>
> 'If I was to pretend that you must take me for what I am inside then that does not work. My body limits it. It is present the whole time. It's not coming to terms with it, an agreed reconciliation. Is it me? I have no choice. It is me, but I am not only it. I have a choice about how I live my life with it. My choice, but the Möbius is constant; everything else is negotiable.'

Talking with a variety of people and ages with Möbius, their need for continuing support becomes apparent. In her influential work in relation to women with breast cancer, Elizabeth Kubler-Ross [1970] developed stage theory, in which the women's reactions to their cancer went through various stages, say of anger, mourning, denial, and then some restoration or reconciliation. These ideas may be useful in acute acquired conditions but for chronic congenital ones they may not be so helpful. Sure, some with Möbius have anger and mourn the faces they do not have; many – most? – children look in the mirror willing their faces to move. But it is a mistake to think that once the child becomes an adult such thoughts pass. For most, as for Celia, Möbius is a daily and continuing presence in the lives.

From daybreak

One person described a typical day in her life and the constraints which Möbius imposes.

> 'When I wake depends mainly on the time of the year. Because my eyes don't close properly, I wake up when daylight comes through the curtains. Getting out of bed is not easy, as my feet tend to seize up over night; managing to stand on them again, find my balance and start walking takes a few moments.

'I often have porridge for breakfast to give me a good energy boost. I need to spend the whole day monitoring my energy levels. If I don't get it right, I can get into trouble quite quickly.

'If I'm going into the office or out to a meeting I like to look good – for me it is very important to make a real effort, put on make-up, do my hair nicely, and wear clothes that are colour coordinated. Just because my face may be a little different from others doesn't mean that I can't feel good about how I look.

'I usually work at home for a couple of hours so I can avoid the rush hour and so get a seat on the train. People very rarely offer you a seat on public transport; one of the disadvantages of having an immobile face is that people probably don't spot that you might be in pain standing up.[2] Standing on a train is not so easy when you don't have much balance, there is always the possibility that I might topple over.[3]

'I live about 6 minutes walk away from the station (for me; others do it far quicker) – because I am unable to drive, it was very important for me to find a home in as accessible place as possible – near to the shops, the station, the cinema, and the bank. It took me about six months to find this place – looking on the Internet, calling estate agents every day and checking how many minutes walk it would take me to get places. My flat is on the ground floor, which makes life much easier. When you have limited mobility, every step matters. I always plan my route for the day very precisely so that I never need to walk more than I can.

'I set off, greet my neighbour on the way out and turn out into the busy street. I pop into the newsagents to buy a paper and have a friendly conversation with the guys there – I pop in nearly every day and we always have a laugh and a joke. I carry on my way when I notice that someone is staring at me. I know it is normal to look at something different or strange and we all do it, but it can be very disconcerting and is invasive of my privacy. The other day, a man stopped me in the street and told me to smile – very unsettling when you can't, and why should I have to explain? It is rare for a day to go by without something like this.

'Crossing roads is tricky; I can't judge how fast cars are travelling, so I often wait ages until I am absolutely sure that it is safe. I get to the station – stairs and unfortunately no lift. I go down slowly and carefully, one step at a time. There is a train there but I won't get to it in time. Other people rush by, but I cannot, I just wait for the next. I get on and find a seat (thank goodness) and we get moving. Some teenagers get on at the next stop – my pet dread. Of all members of the public they are the ones most likely to pick up on my face. I don't want to engage but equally am keen to challenge any assumptions they might be making. I fish out the thickest journal I have in my bag and start to read; maybe they'll see me as the business woman I am.

'I arrive at work and get straight on with the tasks in hand. I love the job, do interesting work, and have great colleagues. I have some people coming in for a meeting whom I haven't met before. This means I'll have to do the full works – lots of body language, non-verbal and verbal, to help them to see me as a person. Wherever I am, whatever context, whether it's meeting someone for the first time professionally, at dinner with friends where there are people I haven't met before, or going to the theatre, I am always conscious that I need to get in first, stop people making judgements based on my appearance and help them feel comfortable engaging with a person whose face doesn't look or work like theirs. I have to convey signals normally conveyed by the face differently, e.g., by the tone of my voice, what I say, making a joke, etc.

'After a couple of meetings, I start to tire (my energy levels are constantly fluctuating during the day) so I eat a banana to help me last until lunchtime. It's hard constantly performing as if on stage.

'I have lots of reading to do – the modern world is full of words – emails, reports, journals, letters, spreadsheets, adverts, papers – and because my eyes don't move reading takes longer and I get lots of eye strain. Wherever possible I try to make the print big and user-friendly.

'I pop out to get some lunch. There's a new guy on the till in the supermarket so I have to make more of an effort – I start talking about the weather, help him see me as a person, not just a different looking face. The afternoon carries on pretty much in the same vein with a constant round of meetings, calls, and emails. I try to work a couple of days a week from home to manage my energy, although pressures on the diary don't always make that very easy. Sometimes I need to have a quick nap during the afternoon just to recharge. Fortunately work is very understanding. It's a constant juggling act with my energy, I have to top it up or it can run down too low.

'My evenings vary, often during the week I might have work commitments, an evening meeting, a reception, or a dinner. If I'm going somewhere new, I plan the route very carefully so I know exactly where I am going. Not being able to see very well makes it difficult finding my way round and, with eyes that are unable to scan, singling out and recognizing people in a crowded place is not easy. Often, when I arrive I stand still and examine the place glimpse by glimpse trying to find the person I'm looking for. Luckily friends and family always look out for me, but if I am networking it's always a bit of a gamble on who I might actually meet. Eating out is another gamble because of my lack of muscles and teeth problems. I always have soft foods – pasta and risotto, and fish, are among the easiest and luckily my favourites too. Steak and most other chewy foods I avoid at all costs. At business events or with people who know me less well this can be embarrassing. I also eat slowly and if I am talking the meal can go on for ages, which I know can be difficult for others if they are in a hurry.

'When I can, I meet up with friends and go for dinner or to the theatre or take in an art exhibition. But I always have to balance these things with taking the rest I can't survive without. Bedtimes never come early enough – and if it's been a busy day it takes time to come down, another Möbius trait with our faulty wiring. So I may not have such a restful night, in part because I am already looking forward to what tomorrow will bring.'

Some with Möbius not only have difficulties in getting to sleep but also have disturbances in sleep, possibly because the sleep areas of the brain, in the brain-stem area, are affected in the syndrome. The problems include interrupted sleep and night terrors in children, which can be an enduring problem for them and their parents.[4] Even in sleep there is Möbius.

Reach out

Children, protected by parents and loved ones, need medical and other interventions. As the child moves out into the world there are other needs, say for assistance with an increasing awareness of difference and with thoughtless teasing and bullying. Teenage years can be bad as friends move on faster and further in love and life. Then it may be wrong to think that adults with Möbius will all have come to terms with and found ways of managing their condition. The early adult years, when leaving the unconditional love of parents, but not always finding a partner or friends, can be as lonely, vulnerable (and in some suicidal) as any.[5]

One woman with Möbius told me that she had a professional group she could call on, as well as friends, including an osteopath, a life coach, and an acupuncturist. Before one disputes the effectiveness of all or some of these groups, this woman is well aware that what she really gains from her support group is the strength to go on, and a reinvigorated sense of self-worth. They also act as a safety net. Both the acupuncture and osteopathy improve her sense of well-being, and she accepts that they help her with strategies and support to go out into the world under her own steam. The life coach, for instance, helped her get back to work once. 'Acupuncture helps me manage my energy and is a real psychological support and strength.' All of these work to maximize psycho-social support, with varying amounts of therapeutic touch.[6]

One might separate health and well-being; one measurable and the concern of mainstream medicine, and the other difficult to quantify but recognized by individuals. Well-being is one area in which complementary medicine is effective, giving time and listening to people's concerns and worries and, through various techniques, bolstering self-esteem in ways in which the busy interventionist and technical medicine cannot always do. Some with Möbius need continuing and varied support throughout their lives, as do we all. Another woman, who was in her thirties, said that the hardest time for her was when her mother had recently died. 'She was the only one apart from me, or even more than me, who had the understanding.'

The UK charity, Changing Faces, has pioneered psycho-social support for those with facial disfigurement. Their methods are multifaceted, from client work including one-to-one support, to groups of people working together on their social skills. Realizing the importance of the social dimension of disability they are also active in school and medical education. They use the media wherever possible, with their Chief Executive regularly appearing on radio and television. They also run poster or billboard campaigns bringing to people's attention the problems of those whose faces are different.

It is difficult to discuss Changing Faces' approach adequately in brief, but the organisation is aware that society makes judgements on people's faces and that these are often critical and damaging to the person, especially someone dealing with low self-belief, sometimes with little support and few social skills. Prejudice of this nature can lead to underachievement, unemployment, and depression.

Changing Faces' main aims in their workshops for clients are to concentrate on three key aspects of poor functioning; self-esteem, social support and social interaction strategies. Put baldly they might sound obvious or even trite. But many with disfigurement have little or no social activity. They need support and step-by-step ideas to overcome their shyness and lack of esteem. One of the important lessons is that these strategies can be learnt.

In a pamphlet, *When Facial Paralysis Affects the Way You Look* [Clarke and Cooper, 1998], strategies are discussed to help those with facial palsy.[7] The social interaction strategies are practical. How do you deal with comments walking down a street, or bullying, or stares? What do you say, think, and do? One time it might be better to ignore comments while another might need a show of assertiveness, without aggression.

The pamphlet suggests that eye contact is crucial, both for talker and listener: 'We look twice as much when listening as when talking. Eye contact lasts around four seconds and can be awkward if more or less.' Normally, this eye contact turn-taking is unconscious, but for those with facial disfigurement it can be so difficult to look another in the face that this breaks down. People are reminded that it is equally bad to be looking too much as not enough. Those with Möbius have little or no blink and so are sometimes accused of staring. Lacking full eye movement, they also have to turn their heads to see someone. So they cannot win; quick glances are difficult, full-on looks are thought to be staring.

Clients with disfigurement[8] are made to realize that people do want to look at people with visible difference but, still, that the main reason people look is to communicate. This can easily be lost in the self-absorption and self-consciousness which follows paralysis when people think everyone is staring at them and self-balance or other balance is lost. Always big on acronyms, Changing Faces uses one to assist here in reducing the space between those with disfigurement and the rest; 'REACH OUT'.

They suggest that the person with disfigurement should make the first, often difficult, move by offering *reassurance*, so inviting the other person to feel less uncertain. The *energy and effort* required to manage social situations is frequently not understood. With Möbius, other people's reactions and the whole conversation must be managed and gauged as it goes along, and without facial expression other channels of communication need to be used. *Assertiveness* at the appropriate time and in the right way is difficult for people with disfigurement but necessary, since merging into the background is not an option. This is hard and some *courage* is required. *Humour* is even more important with disfigurement, since it tells the other person you are relaxed. In the appropriate setting, humour at one's own expense can reduce the distance between people. One man with Möbius campaigned for a student office as 'not just another pretty face' – and won.

Despite all these ideas, there will be still be occasions when things get sticky. Then the person with the disfigurement is asked to focus not on him or herself but on the *other* person, *over there*. By changing the subject, asking open questions about the other person, they might be able to deal with pauses in conversation. The person with the disfigurement has to become a master of the fact that others may not know how to behave; *understanding* may begin with one's own condition but has to involve seeing the other's perspective too. Lastly, and with more than a hint of American self-help manuals and business guru speak, there is no such thing as failure, only feedback. And this feedback has to lead to *trying again*.

Changing Faces also debunks various myths about facial difference. The myths that one can only have a second-rate life with disfigurement, that surgery can fix everything, that the disfigured are brave. They are not; bravery requires choice. The myth of horror films – that looks have any relation to moral character or goodness, of learning difficulties – that those with disfigurement are less intelligent, which is especially a problem with Möbius. Lastly they discuss the myth that appearances doesn't matter – initial judgements are made and looking good and feeling good do go together. Not just looking good, language and attitudes matter too, so with facial difference other streams of communication and expression must be used. They also caution against what is called 'catastrophizing' disfigurement, being made into victims or sufferers, deserving of pity.

Möbius class

Useful though such advice is, Eleanor suggests that Möbius is unlike some other conditions that Changing Faces assists people with.[9]

> 'Möbius is very different to an acquired problem, where the person will have developed with a normally moving face. It is also different from some of the other congenital facial conditions Changing Faces sees. Möbius is not just the face, or the eyes, but the balance, the hearing, etc. It seems almost to have an extra dimension. And because it is there from birth you need to create who you are with Möbius. You have to start without knowing where from.'

Lydia had ideas about how she would give a class in Möbius survival.

> 'I would start by jumping up and down to teach emotion. I would get them to clap hands when happy, stick their thumb up when it's going well. Doing emotion and feeling emotion … you need both. But you need to share, too. When something matters, say moving to my new house, I wanted to tell people and show them, so I went round saying, 'I love my new flat!' to everyone. I could not show it, so I had to keep telling everyone.'

'I don't want to be seen as a disabled person with issues. If one has an internal rage, in the Möbius class, I would teach children to stamp their feet; expressing frustration is important. We don't have nuances.'

James had been unable for years to express his emotions and had felt that the only way to do so was through a breakdown. Similarly, the young woman, Clare, had been admitted to hospital with emotional dyscontrol; unable to express her smaller sadnesses and the frustrations of life she only had huge, explosive ways of expressing. Lydia could understand.

'Not so much now but, at times, I have felt very acute emotion. You go from zero to whatever quickly and you cannot process or assimilate emotion or understand or control it. I learnt to assimilate by experience, and talking, and family. I would teach people how important the cadence and register of the voice can be. A speech therapist came up to me after a conference once and said she had learnt more about the voice from listening to me than she had in 20 years of practising.'

Lydia suggested days out, something originally suggested by Changing Faces.

'We might arrange a day having our hair done, make-up, and have nice things to wear. Then, they would be learning how to make friends, in a context of sharing with others in a similar position. We would do the simple things, which people may not do; go to the pub, go for a walk in a market. We would tackle the big things by doing the small things.

'I would discuss how to start social interactions, by asking questions, say. I used to prepare a list of things to talk about before I went out at university in the evening. It did not come naturally. It was calculated. Being musical is useful, as is any sport; anything as part of a group.'

The aims are to show people with Möbius the importance of non-verbal communication and give them ways of initiating and maintaining conversations without the constant reinforcement of facial feedback.

The attic again

Going to a cinema, or for a meal after work, are at one level of social functioning, but there was another which hung over Matthew, and others: sexual intimacy. Jimmy was struggling with this, too.

'Relationships have been mixed. Sometimes they work and sometimes they don't, though as I get older, it seems harder. You put an ad in the local paper saying 33-year-old, 5'6", blue eyes, salt and pepper hair …

and disabled. What does that mean? If you are trying to sell yourself, how do you go about it?'

Flirting and sending signals are always difficult.

'I am not going to live my life trying to find the right woman. It would be quite nice to find someone, nice to have regular sex, but just not right now. I don't know whether I want to settle down. I quite like being on my own. Maybe marriage is not for me ...'

He is fascinated how people view someone with a disability as a prospective partner. He finds it difficult to approach someone in a bar; he cannot smile across the dance floor – where it may all start through the face. His naïvety does not help; it was not until his late twenties that he had his first intimate relationship. He does wonder what it is to be normal, to be in a relationship, to have children, a mortgage, a dog, and a patio. He has wanted, all his life, to be normal. An online dating service questionnaire asked about eye colour, hair, weight, and height but there was nothing about disability. 'Why isn't there a box for that? Do disabled people not date?'

He decided not to explore speed dating, after all how could someone with Möbius put themselves across in three minutes? On the other hand, many of his friends are still single, so he is not unduly concerned.

Eleanor agreed that it can be difficult to meet people and to circumvent the physical aspect of attraction. Love at first sight is often through the face.[10]

'But if I go back to my late teen years, I was not very embodied as a person and the physical nature of attraction was some way away. I remember a frightening, startling moment when, at a disco, I saw a girlfriend exploring her sexuality and flirting. That was so utterly alien to me. Not because I could not have learnt do it – as I had learnt at university to gossip – but I could not find its meaning. I could not work out what it was about; it had no relevance to me. My friend was fluttering her eyelids and was enjoying herself and you could see the boy and girl doing it. I could not work out why.

'Some do mature later than others but I had not even started. Everything was later. I have friends who got married early; it seemed foreign. I remember when I decided I liked a boy. He didn't notice me, but I was desperate to conform and like someone. It was only at university when I began to know how it all worked but still it did not mean anything.

'At this stage, I did not feel anything physically; even though I had matured physically, I had no feeling. Like the other feelings it had not kicked in. I got it by a gradual process. I had not had really close men in my life and then at university I had close male friends; it helped me find out how friendships worked across the sexes. But even that was confusing because I did not quite know how it worked. When a man was friendly, I didn't know how to interpret it.

'You get there by doing it when it works, by trying, by being prepared for rejection, like anyone else I imagine. This is not just about Möbius. You have things in common; things you like to do together. Then when the time is right, through self-belief and being attractive as a person, as a woman with interests, and your personality, not as a person with Möbius; you learn to take the plunge.'

For her it happened when someone liked her, and liked her for who she was. Then she realized she could be attractive and available.

'OK, I don't kiss like you kiss. Why do you kiss? Because of intimacy, and because it gives pleasure; I do all of that for the same reasons. Even if it does not work like others, it works, you make it work. You have to have the confidence to do it.'

Lydia had managed where some had spent their lives so petrified of failure that in the end they had not been able to try. It is difficult to know whether there are differences between the sexes here. On the one hand, men are supposed to make the first move and so might be at an advantage. But equally men's fear of rejection is huge.[11] Women with Möbius also have an advantage in that they can use make-up, hair, clothes, shoes, etc., to develop their sexuality in ways less available to men. Lydia was also aware that people might seek intimacy for its own sake. How many with Möbius may have had bad relationships just to find someone, and to be loved, even fleetingly?

'There is a risk that, on a physical level, you can go through the motions and not feel anything, carried along wanting physical intimacy alone. You have to be true to yourself. There is a risk, though whether we can say more risk than anyone else, I cannot say. Maybe you'll get thrown back more than others. But by the time you become an adult you will have had so much stuff, that you'll have developed resilience. Underneath I am tough, I have had to be; I need a lot of stuff to be thrown at me before I fall over. And that new man or woman might just be worth it.'

Here the problems are similar in Möbius to those that many have with other facial differences. Changing Faces has workshops on intimacy as well as publishing work in the area. Their approach focuses on typical responses from people with disfigurement. 'Why would anyone find me attractive with my face?'

They discuss how common such thoughts are and try to guide people away from negative thoughts and self-belief and to make them more open and friendly. They give lessons in flirting, when eye contact and body posture are more important than words. Sometimes it just works, as Eleanor related,

> 'That someone can love you with Möbius – be in love with you: that, for me, was the most extraordinary, exhilarating, euphoric moment. It is as though you are completely flooded with happiness. Love is the most completely amazing thing that can be.'

Esprit de corps

Marion Meyerson [2001] asked adults with Möbius how they get by. Members of the US Moebius Syndrome Foundation, they were amongst the higher-functioning and successful people with the condition. She mentions that medical professionals often focus on the physical and clinical problems and the liabilities of reduced or no facial expression. Though important, this inevitably reminds the individual of their difference. She was more interested in the ways in which Möbius might provide strategies for succeeding.

Several things were mentioned again and again and it was striking how many of these are those we all need, whether we live with a condition or not. Family support, faith, and humour are rated amongst the most important. Parents and family allowed Möbians to develop but were also thanked for encouraging people to join social groups, whether church or community groups. Humour was also rated highly, even though without facial expression this is expressed in other ways; people with Möbius laugh when others might smile.

In her book on the pioneering World War II plastic surgeon Archie McIndoe, Emily Mayhew [2004] describes his amazing operating skills and innovations. But, equally, she highlights how he realized that surgery, alone, was insufficient. He encouraged those who he had operated on to mentor and befriend the newcomers, to inform them of what they would be going through. Then, when his patients were shunned in the local town, in shops and pubs, he called a meeting and told the locals that these men, though disfigured, had been injured fighting for their country. Underneath they were just men with the same problems and needs as anyone else. He pioneered horizontal care where patients help each other and the use of education to change society itself, at least in the nearby town.

Meyerson's work highlights the importance of patient support groups for those with Möbius. A number of people were rhapsodic about the Moebius Support Foundation. 'It was life-saving,' 'It provided the missing link,' 'It overcame a sense of isolation,' 'Transformed the pain into an esprit de corps.' Another suggested that it had helped him accomplish, 'What has been the hardest task in life to date – coming to terms with and accepting myself with Möbius.'

Looking back, Lydia agreed,

> 'There is something about being on one's own. I thought I was different, with no one else like me. Even as a little child you realize the world is big and you want to belong. The wonderful work of the support group is beyond praise, the bringing together, the support, whether the camps, or the weekends, they come together and the kids play together and they realize they are not the only ones, there are others looking the same. I never had this till I was 30.'

Similarly Jimmy enjoys helping children in the support group.

> 'You can see yourself in them, and it's great to realize you are not alone. We compare notes, finding out what others do in certain situations, whether it's trying to get a job, get a girlfriend, or how to kiss. Having something so rare, the importance of talking to someone else who understands cannot be underestimated. We have this huge thing in common. I tell them, "Don't let people get you down. If you work at it, it will be OK. I'm not bothered by how many fingers I've got, nor what I look like, just who I am."'

Certainly, it is wonderful to see kids with Möbius playing together, oblivious to the difference they all share, and to see their parents relaxed and able to see a way ahead for once. For adults with Möbius, the continuing mutual support and exploration of their own concerns can also be a lifeline. The various groups have now been meeting long enough that, as children grow into adults, they can share new concerns. Adults can share with kids and their parents, though it is not always easy.[12] Going for the first time as an adult can be difficult too. It was for Lydia, though she accepts that her going was very useful for children and for their parents.

'As an adult you tell the parents, subtly, that it's OK. You model how it can be, show them a life, and a fulfilling one at that, and that one goes on and is happy. How someone can be living a life with Möbius in society, mixing and making friends. You go also of course, so children can see how it works.'

This is where the support groups for those with Möbius, which have become more active over the last few years, are so important.

'It's trying to find a way to be, being you, not just the Möbius. Leading a life, your life, going to the pub, watching the football, whatever. Building self-esteem, just building on Möbius is challenging.'

The politics of Möbius

It was around age 10 that Jimmy's difference hit home. Not only did he look different, he realized, he was different.

'What have I got? Why have I got it? What is Möbius? What can I do to get rid of it …?' He became angry. 'Why him? What had his parents done?' It was so hard to understand. Who could he blame? His loving and supportive parents? If not, then whom? He started to lash out, becoming more and more depressed. In the end, his parents turned to a psychologist for help. After a while he calmed down, bar the teasing and the name calling.

He went from school to college, and ended up at journalist school, finding shorthand a trial, with four out of ten fingers. He went to Los Angeles on an exchange, meeting Bill Clinton along the way. When he returned a friend said how much he admired him for going, 'After all, you are disabled …' Jimmy was taken aback; he no longer felt disabled and shocked that others saw him thus.

After graduating, he wrote at the bottom of his job applications that he was disabled, though since it did not impair his skills he wondered why he mentioned it. Before each interview, he would explain Möbius and it worked for him. Now 33, Jimmy works for a disability support organization. Underneath his coolness there was an anger.

'Just because I am disabled, it doesn't mean I can't have hopes and dreams. Throughout my life I have just wanted to be normal. I pay my taxes, go to work, go for a beer. Just because I am disabled doesn't mean I have to live in my own world. I can walk, go to the gym, post a letter, go sailing and swimming. What is disabling about any of these? It's the culture we live in that wants to identify people's differences and make them disabled … Why can't someone in a wheelchair be a positive role model? It would be nice to see more people with impairments on the television, in a soap opera and not just a token person. I don't suffer from Möbius, I have Möbius.'

Mike Oliver, the UK's first professor of disability studies, who is himself tetraplegic after a spinal cord injury, has written that disability, or impairment, is as much socially induced as medically. Rather than seeing disability as tragedy and 'catastrophized', he suggests it should be seen as difference. Mike has sought to redefine the terms and, more importantly, the perceptions of disability. If disability is seen as a tragedy then disabled people will be treated as passive victims, affecting the way they and others see themselves. Mike and others suggest another model, which has become more accepted and underpins an important document from the Royal College of Physicians of London and The Prince of Wales' Advisory Group on Disability [1992]. In this the following definitions are given:

> Impairment is the loss of abnormality of a particular faculty or part of the body. Someone with a disabling impairment is a disabled person.
>
> Disability refers to a disabled person's encounter with daily living, the environment and society, not only in particular circumstances but encompassing the whole of that experience.

In his book, *The Politics of Disablement* [1990], Mike wrote,

> The individual model [of disability] sees the problem as stemming from the functional limitations or psychological losses assumed to arise from disability, underpinned by the personal tragedy model of disability … Nothing could be further from the truth.
>
> The social model suggests it is not the disability, not individual limitations, which are the cause of the problem but society's failure to provide appropriate services and failure to ensure the needs of disabled people are fully taken into account. Hence disability is all the things which impose restrictions on disabled people, from individual prejudice to institutional discrimination, to inaccessible buildings to unusable transport systems.

Not surprisingly, some have protested that such a model ignores the medical problems which would remain even if all social disability was removed. But for Mike, disability has nothing to do with the physical body and everything about society's inability to support people who are different.

> There can be only two possible explanations why disabled people experience a quality of life so much poorer that everyone else: one that disability has such a traumatic physical and psychological effect on individuals that they cannot ensure a reasonable quality of life for themselves by their own efforts; the other that the economic and social barriers that disabled people face are so pervasive that [they] are prevented from ensuring themselves a reasonable quality of life by their own efforts.

Unfortunately, there are some people with Möbius who find it difficult to maintain an independent life, as we have seen, though it is unclear whether this is because of the pervasive effects of Möbius on their lives, or because of the stigmatization they meet when they go out into the world. The fact that for some their problems began whilst they were very young and still within their family suggests that, for some, Möbius does have a severe, almost suffocating, effect on self-esteem. But for others, it is society's inability to cope with difference that leads to the teasing, bullying, and problems with work and opportunity which Jimmy, amongst others, has railed against.

Mike Oliver is a Marxist, and sees that the reason why society marginalizes the disabled is work. If you cannot produce you have less worth. Yet, while some with Möbius have problems with coordination and vision, rendering them less able to do some jobs, others have no such difficulties and yet have still found job opportunities limited, even when most work now is not manual. This suggests that rather than discounting stigma towards visible difference we should work to reduce its effects. The effects of this are perhaps reflected in that study by Briegel mentioned previously. He found [Briegel, 2006] that behavioural problems in children with Möbius increased when they went to school. Before that, protected by family, their lives were less affected.

Balancing Möbius

Without the personal, subjective accounts of Möbius, this work would have been dry, impoverished, and empty. Equally, though, it is difficult to know if these accounts are typical. For each for whom Möbius remains a barrier between them and the world there may be another for whom it has had little effect. There are successful people with Möbius in the media, in local government, and in many other jobs where their visible difference has made little or no difference. Yet there are also others at home, in their twenties, too paralysed by self-doubt to go out and still dependent on their parents. The people whose narratives have been given are, on the whole, successful and educated, yet still in their inner lives reflect something of their straitjacket.

In a recent postal survey of 21 people with Möbius in Germany Briegel [2007] found a salutary pattern. His sample was aged from 17 to 57 with an average age of 30, and 18 people had been to university. Of these, six had found a partner and three had had children. Fifteen had experienced psychiatric problems, with depression in nine and anxiety in three; of these eight were still having these problems, with six depressed and six reporting suicidal thoughts. Psychometric testing suggested that the men had lower scores in achievement orientation and that the females were more inhibited. As a group they were more inhibited and scored lower for life satisfaction.

Balance is as difficult in such surveys as it is from fuller narratives based on a few individuals. But it is clear that while some find ways beyond their condition, many remain inside Möbius and need assistance in various ways. Whether this is from support within schools, continuing psycho-social support from medical professionals, through the wonderful communities found in various Möbius support groups around the world, or because they meet less stigmatization from others, the hope is for that those with the condition will find more fulfilling ways of living without facial expression.[13]

Chapter 14

The last 'why'

Imagine

Imagine you are a child; but not a child looked back on from your adult perspective and not a child as you once were. Imagine you are a child with one eye which doesn't work, even though it has been operated on. It used to point outwards and though it now looks ahead, it still isn't much use to see out of, so you see one side of the world more than the other. The other eye is not great either, though it is all you have known. But you do realize that it takes longer for you to see things than others, and you don't realize that for most people the world is not fuzzy. In part, you are slow because others move their eyes around to see new things, but you have to move your whole head. Books are one of your loves; they don't mind who reads them and don't mind if you are a bit slow, but sometimes you get dizzy reading, not from the prose but from moving to and fro across each line.

Eating and drinking are difficult; it all comes out of your mouth. This is difficult enough at home but whenever you go out people stare at you eating, and at school some people laugh. You find that tipping the head back is good but the nice speech lady says that is naughty and tries to get you to use your mouth and tongue more. But these don't work well, so you don't really want to. Bits of food get stuck in your cheeks too, and you can't get them out; using the fingers is naughty too; they get smelly and dirty. (Eating and drinking will remain a trial even as an adult. Even when being social, eating and drinking marks Möbius out when you least want it.)

Other kids go to the dentist rarely, you go every holiday and sometimes during the term too. Your teeth are crooked and scaly and need fillings. You don't understand why. Saliva drools from your mouth. You don't care, but it gets sticky and your mother is always after you to use a handkerchief. For her, you do.

At night you lie there with your eyes open. Summers are worse since it is always light when they put you to sleep. You sometimes put a scarf round your head to make it night, but that can sometimes touch the eyes and make them sore, and anyway it is hot and horrid. The eyes get dry and you need drops every few hours. Your mum teaches you to avoid touching them or they get painful and then you need different drops, which sting. Swimming is not easy, what with your mouth always being open and the eyes stinging under water, but with perseverance you learn.

You can't catch a ball and walking over uneven ground or kerbs is difficult. You can't look down and judging distances and speeds is difficult. Then, despite what you do, you are slow and wobbly; others can run and jump but you cannot. Your feet are not springy and your legs don't seem to know how to jump. You practice and practice catching a ball but it never really happens. You don't know whether to give up or not. At school, you are never picked for a team; you hate games and sport and even at playtime; no one says, 'Hi!'

Most of the time, except when you lie in a bath, you can feel your hand and one leg as a constant background nag, which is tiring. You learn later that this is pain. It lets you sleep, but soon after you wake up it comes back. No one asks about it, so you say nothing.

Though you try and try, people find it difficult to understand you when you speak. Your mum and dad are alright, but at school most of the teachers don't understand you, so they always ask the others. You don't mind at one level, since you can just sit there and not be seen, but you also like reading, especially stories. No one asks your opinion. No one wants to talk with you. You love lessons; the teacher lets you alone and you can hide. But you miss a lot of school because of seeing the doctor and for operations. Each time you go back further behind, and no one expects you to catch up. They say you have learning difficulties.[1]

To prove them wrong

Again and again, talking to those with Möbius, they complain of being written off as children, with little or no expectations of success.

If nothing else, this was a potent motivation for Cate, and many others. Others may not have done so well.

Given the sheer number of differing problems that Möbius presents, it is not surprising that its children may need additional support. Celia's childhood was overshadowed, and defined, by the need for attention to her various 'bits' – the body parts she felt so distant from. Gemma's educational achievements are testament to her application and brightness, to the assistance – and persistence – of her parents and to the success of her support workers from surgeons and speech therapists, to teachers, the special needs adviser and teacher for the hearing impaired.

Children with Möbius have been considered to have two intellectual impairments as well as their bodily problems; learning difficulties and autism. Curiously, the prevalence of these two varies hugely between different published series. Learning difficulties were found in 75%, 47%, and 33% by three different groups [Cronemberger et al., 2001; Gillberg and Steffenburg, 1989; Johansson et al., 2001] but only in 5% by Verzijl et al. [2005a] Such large differences need to be explained.

In their thorough work from a mature group of Möbius subjects, 37 subjects with a mean age of 29, from The Netherlands, George Padberg's group [Verzijl et al., 2005a], suggested that there may have been a sample bias in the other studies; one looked at younger people with inadequate testing, and had also recruited by mentioning Möbius and autism, so further skewing their sample. Another studied in a centre for cerebral palsy, again introducing a selection bias and also sampled very young children, under 43 months. Another group took subjects from units concerned with autism, again introducing a bias, and also used relatively poor measures. When these factors are excluded and the tests are applied rigorously, Verzijl et al. [2005a] suggest that there appears to be no learning difficulty associated with Möbius, no reduced IQ, and no deficits in attention or memory. The only cases where there was a learning problem also had autism, to which we will return.

Sample and recruiting bias may be one large reason for an apparently high prevalence of learning difficulty in Möbius, but there are others. The Dutch group, in their understated academic prose, asked at the beginning of their paper if the mask-like face, with crossed eyes, drooling, and speech difficulties, contributed to the assumption of mental retardation in Möbius. They suggest that health care professionals should not presume that limitations in social and interpersonal interaction reflect learning or cognitive problems and in particular that a blank face means a blank mind.[2]

Rhonda Robert, a clinical psychologist, makes the same point,

> 'The physical manifestations of Möbius syndrome contribute to problems in assessment of intelligence, e.g., vision problems, eye movement disturbances, manual dexterity problems, hearing problems, visual–spatial problems, sensory integration deficits, psychomotor problems, motor delay, speech problems, dysarthria, eye movement disturbances, ptosis …'[3]

She goes on to make a plea for care in the administration of various tests in those with Möbius. Their problems with coordination and vision, for instance, may slow them down, especially in tests that are timed. In the Weschler Intelligence Scales, a person who has Möbius syndrome may give an invalid, underestimate of performance IQ because the test needs manual dexterity and visual acuity. 'Future studies need to be designed in which the participants are tested to their strengths.' Remembering Gemma's experiences, as a bright child, having to cope with a multitude of problems while keeping up with her peers in class, one can well imagine that someone with less intelligence may lag behind a bit. The important thing may be to recognize this, provide the necessary support, whether in mainstream or special school, and give each child time. Children with Möbius may be a little slow but their ceiling for achievement is similar to other children.

How many children with Möbius have been shuffled off to schools for those with learning difficulties and physical problems because of their appearance? How many have struggled to escape falsely low expectations? How many still are understimulated, underperforming and misunderstood? Some fight and get there, as we have seen, some have parents ready to fight, but others may not.

Black holes

If learning difficulties are not more common in Möbius, what then of autism? Again published prevalence rates differ, from 5% to 40%

[Bandim *et al.*, 2003[4]; Gillberg and Steffenburg, 1989; Johansson *et al.*, 2001; Strömland *et al.*, 2002; Verzil *et al.*, 2005a]. In continuing excellent studies from Toronto, a figure near the top of this range has been found by Wendy Roberts's group too, looking at young children with Möbius.[5] The high early prevalence might reflect a developmental congenital problem picked up better now than previously. But again another possibility is possible.

The *Diagnostic and Statistical Manual of Mental Disorders: DSM IV* [1994] categorizes people with autism as having impairments in social interaction, communication, and stereotyped behaviours. The social interaction deficits include:

1. Marked impairments in the use of multiple non-verbal behaviours, such as eye-to-eye gaze, facial expression, body posture, and gestures to regulate social interaction;
2. Failure to develop peer relationships appropriate to developmental level;
3. A lack of spontaneous seeking to share enjoyment, interests, or achievements with other people;
4. Lack of social or emotional reciprocity.

The impairments in communication are listed as:

1. Delay in, or total lack of, the development of spoken language (not accompanied by an attempt to compensate through alternative modes of communication such as gesture or mime);
2. In individuals with adequate speech, marked impairment in the ability to initiate or sustain a conversation with others;
3. Stereotyped and repetitive use of language or idiosyncratic language;
4. Lack of varied, spontaneous make-believe play or social imitative play appropriate to developmental level.

Lastly, there are stereotyped patterns of behaviour, interests, and activities. A combination of some of these is taken as support for autism, according to set tests, together with delays or abnormal functioning in at least one of the following areas: social interaction, language as used in social communication, and symbolic or imaginative play.

Impairments in eye-to-eye gaze, facial expression, body posture, and gestures, failure to develop peer relationships, lack of social or emotional reciprocity and language delays: all these cardinal features of autism might have been designed to show the consequences of the embodied features of Möbius. Testing for autism without taking account of the physical limitations consequent on Möbius seems partial and inadequate.

Further evidence of this comes from the different first-person accounts of some of these problems from people with autism and with Möbius. A person with autistic spectrum disorder once told me of her problems with approaching others and looking at them directly [Cole, 1998]. It was, in part, fear, since looking would make people attempt to engage her in interaction, which was a problem both because her fragile sense of self would be, 'Engulfed in a flood of "other"', and 'Because it was so intense an emotional experience as to be intolerable.' In addition, she was not really able to understand facial expression, seeing instead bewildering, complex movements on the face which were beyond her ability to process. She could tell more from a foot falling than from a face. She had married another person with a form of autism; neither of them had looked at each other's face.

In contrast, Celia, wonderfully social and full of fun, had once told me that, 'Twenty years ago I was autistic; you would have thought me so.' She had had very different problems as a child with social activity, which, though they might have given her the appearance of being autistic, were not autistic in nature. For instance looking at another was not a problem. Instead,

> 'I did not know what to do with what they were giving from their faces because I could not give it back. I was flooded with their signals, I understood what they were, but I could not return them. All that communication was one way.'

It must have been immensely frustrating. As I talked, I asked if words might have been a way to reach others.

> 'What you just did with your forehead [I had lifted my eyebrows unknowingly] does not warrant a sentence. If I could have done something back I would have. But facial expressions cannot be translated into words, and even if they could be, as an adult, and not as a child as I was, then the words would take so much longer than the fleeting expressions you make and interpret without really being aware. It is all so rapid and complex and subliminal. I know that now as an adult, and try to compensate, but then I was like a black hole. Things went in but nothing came out.'

The child with Möbius has to contend with multiple physical problems, problems which cut directly between her and others. She lives in a somatic straitjacket, preventing much social interaction and ease of communication. So embodied and deep are these problems that many people have not looked beyond them, not looking inside the chrysalis and giving it sufficient time to develop. Celia developed her social skills over years and lacked the confidence, by her own admission, to become an individual until her late teens and early twenties. For some it takes even longer; some may never have got there, damaged on the way.

In their study, Verzijl *et al.* [2005*a*] found two subjects with Möbius, learning difficulties and autism, but suggested the relationship was solely between learning difficulties and autism, and not between these and Möbius. Though some groups still find an excess prevalence of autism in Möbius,[6] if Padberg's group is correct, agreeing with Celia's reflections, then Alison's Möbius may be completely unrelated to her problems with learning and social interaction. It is a disquieting thought, but maybe we are more accepting of a physical impairment, such as Möbius, being related to learning difficulties than we should be. Along with other lazy, sloppy thoughts, like close-set eyes showing untrustworthiness, or the bad guys looking bad, we are comfortable with there being physical manifestations of mental difficulties. As Wittgenstein wrote [1980], the most difficult thing is to look without prejudice. Put another way, people with Möbius have a social as well as a somatic straitjacket, having to overcome the stigma and low expectations of others as well as their multiple physical problems.

Perhaps some conditions, by the very nature of their impairment, lead to autistic behaviour, even though this does not reflect 'primary' developmental autism (whatever the cause for this). Perhaps this might be recognized in Möbius without a formal diagnosis of autism being made (as in the case in some other conditions). If these are found in a child with Möbius, this should alert people to the problems of the condition and ways to reduce them. Rhonda Robert suggests that such signs should be used to pick up those who need support with the development of social skills and guidance in academic and vocational matters, based on their personal strengths and working around the physical manifestations of Möbius syndrome.

Early days

Perhaps the idea that children or adults with Möbius have intellectual problems will drop away. But this is not to say, given all the problems they have to find a way to reach others and learn about the world, that they do not have additional needs. We saw with Gemma, facing multiple problems, what can be done to allow young "Möbians" to reach their full potential. These problems are complex and alter with age.

Just as at the very beginning of life the face may be of paramount importance to alert people of 'someone home', so the face is also crucial for development in young babies. Babies may not be simply mirroring facial expressions of others but beginning conversations far earlier than was previously thought. Many authors have suggested that mother–infant interactions in the first year of life are important for the conceptualizing of self and object representations and for the early organization of experience. Beebe and Lachmann [1988] provide evidence for early cognitive capacities in babies, with infants a few months old being able to recall patterns and actions for reward. They also suggest that the infant's success in social interactions in the first six months may predict some aspects of later social and cognitive development. These interactions usually develop between infant and mother and are described as being 'dynamic, mutually regulated interplay'; this interplay often focuses on the face.

As Stern [1977] has shown, by two to three months an infant can make and break visual contact with her mother, by looking away and by closing her eyes. By three to four months, this develops into subtle facial expressions of affect. By head movement, mouth opening and closing, and by smiling the infant can communicate slight changes in intensity and quality of mood. Going further, many workers have stressed the importance of 'mirroring' – imitation between mother and child [Beebe and Gerstman, 1980]. Winnicott [1974] suggested that, 'In ... development the precursor of the mirror is the mother's face; what does the infant see when he looks at his mother? He sees himself.' Others have suggested that this mirroring, matching, or mimicry is a key part of mother–infant exchanges in the early months.[7] Detailed analysis of mother infant play at four months has shown that these interactions seem to be controlled not by mother or baby alone but mutually, through very short facial movements of often 0.3–0.5 s. By matching expressions in time and by taking turns in vocalization and gaze, it is suggested that a concept of 'being with' another person emerges.

It may, therefore, be that differences in these early conversations through face, and before spoken language, are the beginning of problems for those with Möbius. It may be difficult for some mothers to interact and stimulate their baby when no facial conversations are possible, where the looping between the two is poorly developed.[8] In addition, the physical problems of feeding, and the need for multiple medical interventions, may reduce the possibility of face play during these early days. Further work may uncover whether a person's success with Möbius in later life reflects his or her early development. Having raised this, however, it is interesting that, anecdotally, the early childhood years are not remembered as being problematic and that behavioural problems in children with Möbius seem to appear later when they meet others from outside their family [Briegel, 2006].

The salience of face

At most meetings I go to, I look around and see, at any one time, round 30–40% of people with their hands against their chins, mouths, or cheeks. This self-exploration may be for reassurance or for a vague simple pleasure. Our body image, our set of thoughts and perceptions and feelings of our embodied selves, seems to have a large facial component.

Children (and many adults) with Möbius seem less aware of their faces; that part of themselves that is relatively passive and unmoving is less salient. Remember Duncan's mother mentioning that, 'He doesn't touch his face as we do during gestures. We had to teach him to feel his face because he was dribbling.'

One of the tasks for speech therapy is to bring into the child's awareness the face as part of what they are, beyond the part which dribbles or has to be tipped back to swallow, as well as to improve speech. People with Möbius sometimes have long journeys to accept their faces.

Understanding and speaking

In discussing the acquisition of speech, one might distinguish speech understanding and speech expression, and suggests that those with motor difficulties with speech acts are likely to be better at receiving and understanding it than making it. But, surprisingly, results from preliminary work in Toronto suggest that those with Möbius may have a greater reduction in understanding of speech than in its use.[9] This has yet to be explained, though Wendy Roberts has speculated that children with Möbius, because of their difficulties in making words and sounds, may not seek out and take part in conversations, so that they are exposed commensurately less to new words and meanings. Those with Möbius, being less social and conversational, may be less available in their crucial early years for the social interactions that underpin and support such learning.

This echoes a debate from the middle of the last century. Jean Piaget [1959] suggested that a child first develops what he called egocentric speech, speech in the presence of other children (and others), and which, though not directed to them, the child assumes is understood by them. This egocentric speech, seen around 3 years of age, is the stream of consciousness or commentator stage as children announce what they are doing and why. He places this in an 'autistic' stage of development, when the child is not aware of others, or herself, as thinking social beings.[10]

He thought that children do not communicate their ideas (before the age of round 7) through social spoken intercourse because, 'The language used in fundamental activity of the child – play – is one of gestures, movements, and mimicry as much as words.' This echoes what Celia said about being more able to communicate with adults, through words, than to her child peers,

> '… with adults, I would have a conversation but with children I was a bystander. Children had another language, a word language, a body language, a facial language. They run around and jump up and down, and I could not do that because my legs did not work.'

The Russian neuroscientist, Lev Vygotsky, challenged Piaget.[11] For him, 'the primary function of speech, in both children and adults, is communication; social contact. The earliest speech of the child is therefore essentially social.'

One of the reasons for the importance of this debate is that if speech development is social and so depends on relationship with others, then any problem with this will affect speech acquisition and development, as may occur in some with Möbius.

Since these ideas were developed over 60 years ago, work has established that language acquisition is earlier and far more complex than was initially imagined. Steven Pinker [1994] discusses work suggesting that babies come into the world with some linguistic skills. In one experiment, one-month-old babies sucked on an artificial nipple with more gusto when given linguistic sounds than nonsense ones. Some infants even come into the world with knowledge of parent's speech; French babies suck harder to French than Russian speech, having heard it in the womb.

Pinker reflects that later, a 3-year-old child is a grammatical genius at a time when he is incompetent at most other things, whether complex theory of mind or social games. He is no doubt as to the veracity of Vygotsky's insight, even likening language to 'another quintessentially social activity', the erotic. He suggests that you need another person to converse with to get language and that you need the other to be interacting appropriately. He cites a time when deaf parents of hearing children were told to let the kids watch TV with the sound up. The children did not learn English. Without knowing the language (and the situation in which words were used) they could not figure it out.

Pinker suggests that, as language is learnt, so our internal thoughts are translated into language in a rather cerebral, though not necessarily conscious, way. But it would seem likely that this mapping may be related primarily to shared action and expression, and in particular through shared contexts; in other words through social interaction, as Vygotsky suggested. For him, words were not disembodied things. This was something to which he returned again and again; 'The meaning within a word was intimately bound up in it ... A word without meaning is an empty sound ... A word devoid of thought is a dead thing.'

He thought that this was one reason why it is so difficult to teach children, because they may learn a word but not its meaning and context.

Many have considered the relation between the development of thought and the development of language, and whether these two are related. In the strongest form of 'linguistic determinism', developed in the early to mid 20th century by Sapir and Whorf, it is considered that our thought is constrained and determined by our language.[12] Vygotsky wrote, 'Thought is mediated by word meanings.'[13] The strongest opponents of this, who include Pinker, suggest instead that thought is independent of the language used to communicate it. People,

> 'do not think in English or Chinese ... they think in a language of thought, [which] presumably has symbols for concepts. Compared with any given language, mentalese must be richer in some ways and simpler in others. It must be richer in that several concept symbols must correspond to a given English word [where there is more than one meaning, e.g., stool] and simpler than spoken language [without] conversation-specific words like 'a' and 'the'.
>
> [Pinker, 1994]

This debate is not yet run, and many people suggest that language does make a contribution to thought, both in adults and during development. It is legitimate to ask how young children with Möbius may develop their thoughts and views of the world when their speech and language lag behind. To communicate their experience and thoughts requires a means to do so, after all. If speech and hearing are difficult it must be so frustrating to be unable to make oneself understood; if the other problems associated with Möbius made it more difficult to assimilate vocabulary and grammar how then might thought develop? Lydia remembers a time of observation and of thought but of no communication, before she had the right words. Matthew once said, 'When I had speech therapy I became a thinker.' Remember Duncan, frustrated by his brothers, saying nothing, calmly waiting hours before smearing their shoes with toothpaste. What was going on in his mind?

'Looking only at the 'g's'

Vygotsky [1986] was clear that the origin of speech acquisition was in social action. Right at the beginning of this process was movement of and between people; gesture. A child may make an unsuccessful grasp of an object, which he called a 'gesture-in-itself'. But then the mother helps the child and the situation changes and the movement becomes a gesture 'for-others', a socially meaningful act; the child then becomes aware that his movement communicates something.

It is not simply during language acquisition that gesture is important. Language and meaning, though we may try to systematize and order it, cannot be confined to such a disembodied logical analysis; language evolved not logically and cognitively but 'in the flow of life that social interaction involves'.[14] Speech, of itself, seems incomplete without gesture; David McNeill [2006] maintains that these two co-evolved and, indeed, are mutually dependent.[15]

> It is profoundly an error to think of gesture as a code or 'body language', separate from spoken language … gestures are part of language. It makes no more sense to treat gestures in isolation from speech than to read a book by looking only at the 'g's.

McNeill approaches language not as words in isolation but part of a thought–language–gesture system, coexisting, codependent, and which unfurls in dynamic temporal sequences. A child of 1 or so will point, and during the subsequent single word period she will point and label an object. Later, when a child combines words together, gestures are reduced for a while but then soon afterwards the number of gestures increases hugely, as they become more refined in relation to meaning. Gesture shows how important it is for language to be embodied, to unfurl not only in speech acts, but in communicative acts within the body, which complement the words and prosody of speech.

McNeill divides communication into a static component in which speech and words have shared meanings and in which language is regarded as an object, and a dynamic one, in which it is seen as a more social, narrative process, and in which gesture acts to give a parallel unfurling imagery component. Gestures and speech are, then, 'Not only communications but ways of cognitively existing, of cognitively being at the moment of speaking.'

Many with Möbius have small or non-existent gestures. I asked Celia about when she could not respond to people around her with speech, why she did not try gesture. She replied,

> 'I did not have gesture because I had not learnt it.'

Normally we don't learn it, it just appears, I suggested.

'But I did need to learn it. All my gesture is voluntary, even now aged 46. Everything I do, I think about … All the things I am doing, whether turning my head or moving my hands, is all self-taught. I learnt from observation as an adult. I had some, crude, version as a child and teenager. I had the words, but words are not appropriate. Your face is doing a load of different things. Without that, what can I do?

'When I was a child I could not gesture, because I was a collection of bits. My body was not me, so expression in it, with it, would not be from me either. It was not a joined-up feeling. There was huge bit missing; with the lack of balance, mobility, and problems with coordination, you don't get a sense of self … I could see everything and wanted to communicate but I could not do anything. It makes you so different. The adults may have been trying hard but I could not give back.'

Celia, a Cartesian child trapped in her head, had thoughts and words but no facial expression or gesture. Without this she could talk with adults in big talk, about literature and hospitals, but had no small talk and no way to communicate much of her experience.

Right before you

In the last chapter of my book, *About Face*, I developed a theory of why the face evolved (or at least I thought I developed a theory; one colleague called it my 'random stream of consciousness' chapter). Humans are the only species with such a developed mobile expressive face. I suggested that it evolved as we became more social and needed to attend to, and understand, our peers more. With the development of more complex and subtle emotions, in a more complex and subtle social world, there needed to be an embodied expression of these inner states. When we converse with someone, we usually look at their faces not only to watch the mouth move, though this does affect speech perception, but for the rapid movements of the face, which add expression to the words and the gestures.

Communication is, therefore, not simply through speech, not through speech and gesture but through speech, gesture, and facial expression, with each adding in overlapping ways: speech, meaning in a codified agreed system; gesture, a more dynamic social imagery; and facial expression, an affective dimension. Sometimes, these will be in harmony, all adding to a single thought or communication, sometimes they work in more complex, complementary ways, an embodied symphony of meanings. And, of course, each channel does not do a single thing and, together, the channels may give differing messages. In irony, for instance, words may say one thing, the tone of voice, gesture, and facial expression another. Interestingly, one man who had 'temporary Möbius', due to bilateral facial nerve paralysis, found that it became crucially important for him to be clear and unambiguous in what he said in order to communicate; without moderation through facial expression, shades of meaning were lost.

So communication usually involves words, prosody, facial expression, and gesture all working dynamically in various ways to create a whole. Lose one and you might think that all would not be lost. But without facial expression, as in Möbius and from birth, and with a withdrawal from or lack of development of a feeling of embodiment, then the consequences may be severe.

Children learn not only to communicate their own thoughts and needs, but learn about others, and that these others possess mental states like them. This development of a 'theory of mind' usually takes place around 4 to 5 years old and enables a child to gauge others' beliefs, desires, and intentions and so become social and interactive, listening to others as well as communicating needs and wants [Baron-Cohen, 1994]. Autistic children are known to have deficits in this, but so have other groups. Jean Lundy [1999] reviews briefly work on deaf children and their delays in theory of mind.

The deaf children of hearing parents can be delayed in the development of mentalising, though deaf children of deaf parents are not. There is evidence that when hearing mothers interact with their deaf children, communication about mental states is rare. Deaf children may get less explanation for feelings, attitudes, and reasons for other people's actions and, if they have less exposure to discussions about mental states, they may have deficits in their vocabulary of mental processes and in their development of theory of mind (in a weak Sapir–Whorf manner). In turn, children with an immature theory of mind are slower to understand about others' mental states, and this may result in deep and long-lasting problems in understanding people, social events, and interpersonal relationships.

There is no work as yet on the development of this mentalising in young children with Möbius, but given their other problems, such work would seem timely. With hearing and speech problems, as well as lagging behind in socialization for a number of reasons, it may well be that children with Möbius are not exposed to as much social speech, leading to further problems. Intriguingly Lundy concludes her short article by suggesting that,

> 'Children's literature may be especially useful for theory-of-mind development in deaf children. By reading to children, teachers expose children to alternate views of the world. Stories provide an opportunity to free children from confinement in the present and what can be immediately seen and touched, and lead them to a world beyond everyday experience.'

As we have seen, many children with Möbius become avid readers, to learn about the world and reach out beyond their condition, and continue to be so into adult life.[16]

The last 'why'

Facial expression is not just a peri-linguistic add-on; it helps reveal inner states of feeling not accessible through other channels. And these states are not peripheral in our actions and activities of daily living. Vygotsky [1986] wrote that:

> Thought is not begotten by thought; it is engendered by motivation, i.e., by our desires and needs, our interests and emotions. Behind every thought, there is an affective–volitional tendency, which holds the answer to the last 'why' in the analysis of thinking ...
>
> To understand another's speech, it is not sufficient to understand his words – we must understand his thought. But even this is not enough – we must know its [affective–volitional] motivation. No psychological analysis of an utterance is complete until that plane is reached.

As we have seen, some with Möbius have reduced experience of emotion, to the extent that it is an unknown category to them, at least in their early years. Why?

In 1948, Ruesch described patients with psychosomatic problems as being unimaginative and showing difficulties with the verbal and symbolic expression of emotion [Ruesch, 1948]. Later, Sifneos [1972] called this alexithymia, meaning the inability to express feelings with words.

These patients also tended to have 'constricted emotional functioning', a poverty of fantasy, and an inability to find appropriate words to describe emotions. Alexithymia has been divided into primary, an enduring impairment, like a personality trait, and secondary, which is usually a reaction to severe psychological trauma. Within these ideas it is not entirely clear whether emotional language and expression and emotional experience itself can be clearly separated. In relation to Möbius syndrome, alexithymia may be a label rather than an explanation. One person with Möbius, when I mentioned this term to her, suggested that her psychological trauma must have been before birth.

One explanation for the emotional problems seen in Möbius might be that the primary brain problem, in the brainstem area, could be associated with loss of emotional circuits or neurotransmitters related to emotion too. Imaging studies might be designed to assess this. But not all those with Möbius volunteer this loss, and the fact that those without emotion as children can develop it later, suggests that such a primary, congenital emotional deficit may be unlikely or, at least can be reversed.

More recently, echoing Vygotsky, Antonio Damasio [1995] has drawn attention to how emotions underpin our lives. Patients with frontal-lobe damage, who may have reduced or even absent affective perceptions, for instance, may have normal intelligence and memory, but find it difficult to get by from day to day. They cannot make decisions, since those require information about the alternatives and an emotional steer one way or other.

Damasio differentiates between emotions – inner mind states – and feelings – their expression in and on the body. Feelings, in turn, might be closely linked to emotional experience. Thus, basic emotions like anger, happiness, and fear, are felt when the face and autonomic body conforms to the patterns for such a state. More subtle emotions, wistfulness, euphoria, for example, are tuned by experience and combine central emotional and cognitive states with subtler feelings in the body. Lastly, he suggests, there are bodily feelings of which we may not be aware. In this model, feelings are felt in the body and the face and fed back to the brain, to be elaborated into emotional experience.

Feelings are sensors for the match or lack thereof between nature and circumstance. Feelings, along with the emotions they come from, are not a luxury. They are the result of a most curious physiological arrangement that has turned the brain into the body's captive audience.

Damasio [1995]

In this elegant prose, Damasio echoes the work of William James and of the Danish psychologist, Carl Lange, who suggested that the conscious experience of emotion was secondary to its bodily, physiological emergence. Consider our response when we see a snake. We jump back before we feel scared; the feeling follows the action for such rapid, intense experiences. James wrote, 'We feel sorry because we cry, angry because we strike.'[17] And, one might add, happy when we smile. Though this may explain some short severe and rapid emotional responses, it is also clear, as Damasio suggested, that some feeling states last longer than their trigger and some may have a less clear relation to bodily feelings. Emotions may drive our long-term actions; some evolutionary psychologists even suggest that love is designed to pair-bond long enough to bring up children.

The emotional problems of Möbius might therefore reflect the absence of embodied expression of emotion, in Damasio's terms due to a deficit in bodily feelings and in particular in feelings from the face. As that young boy asked, 'Why can't I be happy?' Without facial expression the emotion was absent too, he reasoned.

Fridlund [1991] reviewed the evidence for this 'facial feedback hypothesis' and found none of it convincing. He used examples, however, which were necessarily limited: Bell's palsy, in which one side of the face is paralysed, and drug-induced temporary muscular paralysis. Neither provided evidence for changed mood and emotion following reduced facial movements, but both were unusual situations and unlikely to reflect natural functioning.

Adelmann and Zajonc [1989] were much more convinced, and quoted experiments in which subjects posed emotion whilst looking at a scene or film and rating it as sad or happy. Those posing a smile rated the film funnier than those posing a grimace. In one ingenious paper the subjects viewed a cartoon with a pen in their mouth, either between the lips, (so preventing smiling), or between the teeth, (so enabling, even facilitating, smiling). The latter group found the film funnier. All such studies have many drawbacks, not least that a posed smile is hardly natural, but it is possible that there may be a contribution to central emotional experience from facial movement that is unavailable to those with Möbius.

Any deficit as a consequence of the absence of facial movement might have a more subtle cause too. Pinker described thought in mentalese, in a rather cognitive model. But there is evidence linking perception and action. Recently Simone Bosbach et al. [2005] studied two subjects without any perception of touch or movement sense below the neck. This led to severe problems with movement: these subjects have limited movements, which they have to think about and monitor visually. Importantly they have also lost skilled automatic movements. They were asked to view a series of videos of actors picking up boxes of differing concealed weights and then decide two things. The first task was to decide how heavy each box was (they were told that there was a small series of boxes of different weights), and in this they were normal. But in a few trials, the actors were given wrong information about the weight in the box. The two subjects were then asked to judge not the weight, but what the actor's expectation of the weight was. In this they were much worse compared with control subjects. The authors suggested that the subjects with sensory loss were deficient because, to make judgements about expectation in another, they needed access to their own subconscious internal programmes for movement and these, it was argued, might be deficient because of their condition. In other words, to make some perceptual judgements you need, at some level, to imagine performing that act.

Some years ago Andy Calder [2000] led a series of experiments on how well a small group of people with Möbius could recognize the facial expressions of emotion in others seen from carefully selected photographs. The subjects with Möbius were normal in this; to recognize facial emotional expressions you do not need to be able to move the face. But then they asked the subjects to describe what the face did when various emotions were displayed; how does the mouth move in sadness, or the eyebrows in surprise? In these tests, those with Möbius did show deficits, though the sample size was too small for this to be statistically significant and so this was not part of the paper. But, if confirmed in larger samples, it suggests that internal programmes or models of facial movement may be accessed and necessary to describe facial expressions, and that without these models the ability to imagine and describe is reduced.[18]

This raises the possibility that another reason for reduced emotional experience in Möbius may be that this relies not only on bodily feelings of facial movement but also on central stored models of these movements, which presumably are not developed in Möbius. Vygotsky wrote of language being internalized once it was learnt, so we could think without speaking. Wittgenstein [1981] asked, '... Do you look into *yourself* in order to recognize the fury in *his* face?' Maybe emotional experiences are somewhat similar; as children we express and find the boundaries for expression whilst later, some emotional experiences may be internalized by employing, at a subconscious level, the same programmes used in bodily expression of emotion.[19] Without having made facial expressions of emotion, those with Möbius lack the internal motor programmes the rest of us use, without knowing it, when internalizing emotional experience.

Looping

Thus far, we have considered the causes for impoverishment of emotional experience in rather singular, impersonal terms. People with Möbius might find emotional experience difficult because they have not had feelings in the body, and because without programmes to make the emotional acts on the face they find it difficult to internalize emotion. And without feeling an embodied being, as Celia described, other channels for emotional expression, like gesture and posture and action, which are pre-eminent in children, might be unavailable too.

Yet, right from the beginning, a child is not alone but in relation with others; we are social not solitary beings. And this leads to a further reason for emotional impoverishment. Without embodied expression of emotion, on the face, in gesture, in how we move, the possibility of emotional communication with others is reduced.

Beebe and Lachmann [1988] discuss the relation between facial and other behaviour and the infant's inner experience. At early ages, the infant's observed actions are assumed to parallel her experience, then by 6 months or so, actions and inner experience may not always be always similar. Mother and child may influence each other in matching timing and affective facial behaviour to know something of the other's perception and feeling state. As empathy develops, they suggest, facial and other behaviour may become similar; matching facial behaviour can lead to generation of similar feeling states themselves. Paul Ekman [1983] provided evidence, before the discovery of mirror neurones within the brain, that the mimicking of certain facial expressions by actors can produce similar autonomic changes in heart rate, etc., as are seen in the person making the original facial expression. Matching facial expressions may, therefore, match physiological states that might be felt, and so add to the emotional matching between people.

Without embodied, readable, emotional expression in voice, in facial expression, in gesture, we cannot extend our feelings to others and are not available for the emotional conversations between people that underpin our social and emotional lives. Merleau-Ponty wrote [1964b] that, 'I exist in the facial expression of the other as he exists in mine.' Faces do not just feed back to their owners, they are designed and have evolved to be seen by others and we gauge our social success by how others treat us. Perhaps emotions are expressed socially by children, as they use others' responses to them to gauge the acceptable use of such expression. Then, as they develop, emotional expression may become internalized more, so that as adults, depending on our culture, we may remain stiff-upper-lipped as our wives run off with a car salesman, or England lose the cricket to Australia once more.

We normally become accomplished whilst young, without ever being quite aware of so doing; in contrast, Lydia and Eleanor had to study and learn it consciously in their teens and beyond. They aped gesture, they learnt social speech, gossip and then, through gesture and prosody of speech, became social and emotional. They bootstrapped embodied emotional expression into internalized emotional experience, without facial expression, by imbuing gesture and prosody with meaning and feeling and in so doing by reaching to others in a manner unavailable to them as children.

James, Celia, Cate, Eleanor, and Lydia, all discussed their reduced emotional experience, especially as children. Fortunately most gained such experience later in their lives: some did this through classical music,[20] whilst for others, like Lydia, rote learning of gestures from others began the transformation, to be followed by immersion in a culture where emotions were within gesture as much as within facial expression.

This suggests how important it is to give emotional experience to young children with Möbius, through any available means. One family with an adolescent boy talk their emotions and feelings the whole time, encouraging him to do the same. At a recent scientific meeting on Möbius there was a session on treatment, and the discussion ranged over dentistry, speech therapy, eye surgery, etc. But others were arguing for psycho-social support for the children and their parents, and that made the point that this support may be needed lifelong. But it also seems vital to drag young children into their bodies and so into a social world. Perhaps body brushing has some effect by making children aware of their bodies more. Perhaps physical as well as psycho-social interventions – anything that encourages connection between mind and body – are needed to prevent further Cartesian kids. Any movement that drags Möbians out of their head and into their bodies will bring them closer to the world and closer to others.

'The word is stronger ...'

Fortunately, many with Möbius do get emotion and feeling. Though they do not smile with their faces they do with elsewhere, with shrugs of the shoulders and with laughter. In fact, when together, a group of Möbians are laughing and shoulder heaving a fair amount of the time; so much so that one wonders if they have developed a shared sign language for emotion. But this is not to say that the emotional expression and world of Möbius becomes similar to everyone else's. Lydia once more:

> 'With Möbius you have to be much more wordy and articulate and this requires intelligence and so it can be hard and tiring. I am articulate but also interested in language, so I can use words to express what I am feeling. Say, in a relationship, I am more likely to use words for reassurance that

I am picking up the right signals. For me the word is stronger than facial expression.

'Without the word, how to express the feeling? When I played the piano, it helped me to reflect my feelings. When I teach language, I teach total physical response. So, certainly we talk about non-verbal. What I am interested is the non-facial and some of that is gesture and tone of voice. Gesture is part of language, is a language, and people with Möbius do not always learn it; they must be taught.

'Without gesture, thought is impoverished, as is language without gesture and thought without language … I learnt gesture as well. It makes language much clearer for my audience and for me. I use sign language as something for emphasis. To ask children to shut up, then, you go, 'Shush.' as well. We have conversations in angry voices or quiet voices, this makes it far fuller so I was then feeling it too. Use the hands and you feel it too.

'As a child, I did not know I was missing out. To reach out to others, I needed embodied expression – feeling. As you grow up, the social feedback from others has far more meaning than as a child. A meaningful smile from you triggers an emotional response from me. As a teenager, I was articulate but this was insufficient. I had words, I read, I was eloquent: I could talk to adults, they could understand me, but none of this helped with my fellow teenagers.

'How did I develop me? I got on with it, with what I've got. It's not about liking it, but it is certainly assuming the physical and putting it into the mix. As a child, I developed things I liked doing. I didn't do the horse riding, but read books and did piano instead, so I was becoming a person. I became an adult young because I couldn't do childhood. I did choose to be who I am, starting with a blank slate. I was also a bright child and I have always analysed and reflected. I realize that to have Möbius and a learning problem must be far more difficult. Being clever allows more ways out. My greatest opportunity is my brain, but it can also be harder since you mind so much more and a wider perspective can be worse. I know a girl with Möbius who drives, goes clubbing, and works in a shop; her life may be easier.'

Emotional catch-up

Damasio wrote of basic and more subtle emotions and of bodily feelings, of which we may or may not be aware. Sitting with Lydia, richly emotional and aware of her inner feelings, as well as keeping a trained eye on yours, is stimulating and enervating. Like Vin talking of Cate, there are few dull moments; having developed emotional experience later in their lives they seem always to be exploring theirs, and yours, and articulating much of their feelings. It is as though they dip into the basic, the subtle, and the bodily feelings and are constantly aware of them in a heightened and enriching way. With them, there is no numb zone, no emotional deadening but rather a life-affirming presence, without facial expression but with gesture, with bodily expression, and with a keen intelligence exploring and relishing their feelings and yours.

Stimulating though this can be, Celia discussed some of the consequences of becoming more attuned to her and others' emotions.

'I think that I rely on the social feedback more, because the embodied is less present. This makes me very vulnerable to other people's states of mind, whether angry, sad, or happy. I pick up signals and it can be very unsettling for me. I have to do something to myself to remind myself that it is their stuff not my stuff. I have found that very hard and only recently have I found a way which works for me. Otherwise I can be caught up in another's situation.

'It is very difficult to describe the energy I need. It is exhausting, even just talking to you now. Walking is an effort; sitting on my own, doing nothing, is not. But as soon as I start exteriorizing myself it is an effort, because I have to think about gesture and about what I think about. I always know what I am going to say. If I don't know the end of a sentence, then I slow down. It's not natural with Möbius. Tiredness is a constant thing.

'I do the full-on much of the time; at work and in front of people, always full-on. It is effort or you are a wallflower. It is very tiring to manage the social the whole time. Still, after all these years, every time I meet someone I am managing how they perceive me, how I can try to help them, how I can help them if they don't know me, how they might be shown how to respond. Any person with a disfigurement has to manage each social interaction they have and if this is done badly this can lead to negativity. I have to manage all this without the other people realizing each day, all day, every day.

'In spite of having a heavy bag to carry about, you can still live and enjoy. It is frustrating when people don't know just how heavy it is.

'Living is a daily marathon to be thinking about so much and sometimes the energy is not there. I manage my week to order things I do, so I have quiet and less quiet days, some face-to-face, some at home on the phone. I can never just get up and not have to have things planned. There is no spontaneity; that cannot work. I am forever arranging things and then having to cancel at the last minute. I feel I am letting people down.

'But there is also something about the intensity. When I get nervous, it is very sharp and intense and I cannot control or gauge it the same. Because I don't have the mechanism within the body to control it, I cannot cool down emotionally. If too excited, then I can't sleep. I cannot calm myself down.'

Even with emotion then, its communication 'exteriorization' appears more intellectual, and tiring. But neither Lydia nor Celia would go back to how they were. Lydia:

> 'When I was playing emotional catch-up I never associated that with Möbius. Now I am happy most of the time but I started to be happy at university. Before that, external things made me happy, if we went to a play or I read a nice book, but it was things making me happy. Only as an undergraduate did happiness come from me. An emotion is what you feel, a state of mind, what you think. If it's a nice day you can think that's a nice day, warm blue sky, green grass, nice view, etc. and you can think happy … but to be happy – an emotional experience – you have to feel it. Sometimes I feel happy and I smile on my face but you don't see it.'

When we were talking, Matthew had also discussed his distinction between emotional feeling and expression.

> 'Happiness is an internal concept and has nothing to do with the smile. A smile is a symbol of happiness. Real happiness is ephemeral, like catching a butterfly. I would not even say in the brain because it is within the whole person, within the heart and the soul. If I am happy it is because I am satisfied with what has happened and this validates me.'

Lydia continued.

> 'I know I get that smiling happiness thing from you but you don't get it from me. I was thinking recently, perhaps because I don't give people any they, in turn, don't give me any.'

Celia said a similar thing:

> 'When I express being happy that has to be vocal and intellectual … There is an element of artificiality of the expression but not the feeling. Even with emotion now, I have two sorts of happy, intellectual happy to express, and happy happy. I can be happy, not think happy, but to express, I have to think. When I do too much I don't feel good, slightly sick, slightly giddy and sluggish.'

Emotional experiences are not, of course, confined to happiness. After a relationship ended,

> 'I cried for a year, every day. I think I was crying for everything that had happened, not necessarily about my lost relationship. It was not therapeutic; it was way too painful. It was a vehicle for expression that I had not had before; it was a year I mourned both my lost and new-found experience.'

Another with Möbius who had developed emotion as an adult also described how occasionally she would feel the wrong thing. For instance, when seeing a sad scene she might want to laugh. It is as though the emotional bootstrapping she had learnt was at times misdirected. Fortunately this is infrequent and easily concealed.

Meyerson [2001] has discussed the possible consolations of Möbius. Several of her correspondents were keen to celebrate the accomplishments of those with Möbius as well as their problems and for many these included pushing themselves that bit harder. Having lived through teasing and rejection, many thought they were more sensitive and compassionate and many work in areas where they meet others professionally, whether in medicine, counselling or teaching.

Eleanor agreed, and then described her own philosophy.

> 'Möbius has given me an ability to see things and judge them and value them more. I don't get fussed by little things, only the big things. My piano this week would not fit through the door. So? Having not had friends as a child, having operations, etc., something now has to be really bad for me to be worried about it. I get worked up now but only about the big things.
>
> 'Möbius has taught me to value the simple things that make you happy. Don't wait for dreams to come true; value the nice book, or walk, or a shared meal. That makes me more grounded and stable and I think I get more pleasure on a daily basis. In fact I think I am happier each day than my friends because I have known the pain of isolation, etc. After 15 years of life without having a giggle or a conversation or not going to cinema because you have no friends, then everyday is a pleasure. Möbius has made me who I am today.'

We can all see bad teeth or a club foot and know these need help and treatment. We can correct eye misalignment and, though this is largely cosmetic, allow the person to appear less different. But how many of us know what it is like to meet new people each day who stare or move away? And how many of us know what it is like not to feel? Face and social interaction, face and self-esteem, face and feeling; being inside Möbius is extraordinary and almost unimaginable. Those who live with the condition allow us all insights into what our mobile, expressive face does by showing us something of life without it.

Postscript: Duncan, grown up

I had first met Duncan 10 years before when he was around 12, though then I had spoken mainly with his mum. It was clear that Duncan had some problems with emotional expression and experience, since he appeared not to have been excited at Christmas or on his birthday. I returned to find out how he was now as a young adult. This time I chatted with both Duncan and his Mum.

When Duncan and his parents went to their first Möbius conference, in his late teens, his Dad said, 'We shouldn't be here.' One can understand this, since Duncan's Möbius is less noticeable than many. Speaking with him one might not notice, since he has limited movement around both the lips and eyes, though above his eyes the immobility is more pronounced. In favour of Möbius is his lack of eye movement laterally. But, overall, Duncan does not think it affects his day-to-day life at all. This reflects both its mildness but also his other problems.

He has arthrogryposis, a congenital stiffness of the joints, rendering his fingers stiff and unbending, and his legs inflexible.[21] He also has a form of spina bifida, picked up a little late, which explained his lack of concern about soiling his nappies as a baby; he could not feel there. He has worn a back brace for several years, but occasionally still collapses and is unable to get himself up, feeling weak and then stiff.[21] He can spend a day or so recovering from an attack lying helplessly in bed. He also has some insensitivity to pain. Once he had a dart stuck through his hand, pinning it to a table. He just asked his Dad what to do. His Dad pulled it out, washed the wound and rang the hospital. They said that was enough, so they just carried on, though the darts game was over. He has burnt the skin off his hand, smelling the injury rather than feeling it.

Möbius, then, is not such a big deal. But then it is also all he has known, it is his normal. He does not remember speech therapy, though his Mum does well. They had to start again when his milk teeth fell out and no one could understand him. He had learnt to speak using his teeth as a front stop instead of his lips.

He still does not get excited much. In his own words, he just accepts things as they come along.

> 'If someone does something wrong to me I don't know if I feel anger; I don't kick things or hit them, I just don't feel like doing that ... I don't get stressed out, I tend to withdraw onto my computer, with its music and graphics. I don't know what I would do without music. I like hip hop and club stuff and mixing. I like listening to the lyrics; I listen and understand the situation and them explaining what it is like on the streets.'

Listening, and then thinking, allows him to understand others. I mentioned James telling me that he thought he was in love and only later felt it. Duncan understood.

> 'It's not that I want to do music, it's because I miss it if it's not there. I have a few good mates, but I don't need to see them lots, as long as they are there for me. I switch off if I've had enough of whatever outside. I have more social life online than elsewhere.'

He also likes graffiti, and once got arrested with his mate as they sprayed paint over a wall. His mate was covered in green paint while Duncan was caught red-handed, literally. 'No real point denying it.'

His partner Siobhan finds Möbius difficult. They met on the Internet. Though they had been going out for some time, it was a slight surprise when their son Archie was born a few months ago. Duncan does not talk about his feelings about this.

> 'It's not that I don't want to: I have nothing to say. It's just me, sometimes there's nothing there. I argue with Siobhan and she says leave, so I just pack my bags, and then she gets angry because I have not fought to stay.'

Though he cannot recognize feelings, he says, he has always found things humorous 'in a way'.

> 'If I find things funny, it is not to say that I am happy. If someone dies, I switch off. I don't really have different moods. If someone stresses me out I tell them and then move on. Do I ever feel fed up? I don't know. At a funeral, I just do what the others do [rather than feel].'

I thought of Lydia learning at university to mimic action and gesture socially without taking it within her.

He is now helping to run a website for hip hop lyrics and graphics. He started by logging on and kept complaining when people broke the site's rules. They picked up on this and asked him to help, and now he is almost in charge. Though the owner lives a few miles away, they have never met. He is online most of the day, and has made nearly 7000 hits in the last year.

He finds it easy to write lyrics, which others appreciate, without feeling what he writes. The words pour out and only later might he understand them. He finds the site peaceful. He has written stories about a sniper, about a polar bear, and many others. 'I can put myself in the stories.

I think I know what they are feeling more than what I am feeling.' He spends so long on the laptop that once Siobhan threw it across the room. 'She watches TV. I do this. When I am talking online it is me, when I am writing and doing graphics I am somewhere else.' His writing has won rap leagues and tournaments, again judged online.

With the graffiti and some of his other pranks, involving breaking a few windows of his old school, he says he likes risk. For that reason he admires the talented graffiti artist, Banksy. But then I asked him whether he worried about what might follow from his risky actions. For the most part, he did not, so the risk was lessened. He had never been big on consequences.

But now, he said, if he were to go to prison, there is a consequence; Archie needs to be cared for. 'He is a commitment, like family.' I hesitated to say he was indeed family. I ask what happens when Archie, who was gurgling happily from a mobile baby chair on the mat, gives Duncan a great big smile.

> 'Seeing him smile, I enjoy it and share it like no one else. I share his pleasure. When he smiles I smile, on the face [a bit] and inside. I am upset when he is upset.'

He may only be 15 months old, but he is already teaching Duncan how to feel.

Notes

Chapter 1

1. Möbius syndrome is often written in English as 'Moebius'. In German its pronunciation is approximate to 'Muh-bius', with a short first syllable. In England people usually say 'Mee-bius' whilst in the USA it is often pronounced 'Moby-us'. We will spell it as in German, though many references use the anglicized spelling.

2. Josh's observation suggests that he was aware of the facial expressions of those around him and of their relation to inner emotional states he has no direct experience of himself. This will be considered in more detail in later chapters of the book.

3. Here we are using the terms 'feelings' and 'emotions' in a similar way to Damasio [2000], with feelings experienced as if in the body and emotions more in the brain. But such a Cartesian separation between mind and body, it is accepted, is deeply erroneous and difficult to defend, and used only in the hope of it being a useful approximation.

4. From the introduction of Harriëtte Verzijl's (excellent) doctoral thesis. [Verzijl, 2005].

5. [Möbius, 1888] As Verzijl suggests, Möbius is remembered for his syndrome, for an ocular sign of hyperthyroidism and for a description of ophthalmoplegic migraine. His work on the weak-mindedness of women and the pathology of men of genius seems to have aged less well.

6. This is adapted from the classification of Towfighi *et al.* [1979].

7. The first scientific meeting on Möbius was held in Bethesda, Maryland in the Spring of 2007, organized by Vicki McCarrell and the US Moebius Syndrome Foundation.

8. Ventura, L. Environmental and teratological factors – hypoxic and vascular events; misoprostol and other known teratogenic agents, *Moebius Syndrome Scientific Conference*, Bethesda, MD, April 2007.

Chapter 2

1. Many children must have died with Möbius in the past because of feeding problems.

2. The Moebius Syndrome Foundation, c/o Vicki McCarrell, PO Box 147, Pilot Grove, MO 65276. www.ciaccess.com/moebius/

3. Laughter is different in Möbius without the facial clues and without the wide opening jaw. Möbians tend to have a higher laugh but also often lift their shoulders in compensation.

4. The mother of one boy with Möbius said he was such a good boy, meaning he was not naughty, or spirited, as a child.

5. There is a similar statement of love and defiance, devoid of concern about difference, in Gabriel García Márquez's *One Hundred Years of Solitude*: 'If you bear iguanas, we'll raise iguanas.'

6. Such an idea has far more widespread acceptance now. It is, for instance, known that children born without limbs can have phantom limb sensation of that missing arm or leg; the perception of the limb appears hard wired and innate.

Chapter 3

1. Cleft palate and high arched palate are two of the comparatively rare craniofacial 'malformations' associated with Möbius syndrome. In a Dutch study, 10 out of 35 people with Möbius also had some degree of hearing loss [Verzijl *et al.*, 2003].

2. Small jaw or micrognathia is another common associated problem. Verzijl *et al.* 2003].

3. Aged 6, she had blocked tear ducts and her eyes streamed constantly. Another operation followed.

4. A similar discordance between language comprehension and expression has been found in a series of Möbius children in Toronto. [Wendy Roberts, *Moebius Syndrome Scientific Conference*, Bethesda, MD, April 2007].

5. A competent and dynamically functional closing valve or sphincter between the nasal cavity and mouth and throat is essential for normal eating, normal breathing, and intelligible speech. In a pharyngoplasty, a sphincter is positioned between the oral and nasal cavities and coordinates appropriate airflow through each chamber to allow a better voice. The sphincter also prevents nasal regurgitation during eating and allows pronunciation of consonants, while opening the port can improve respiration.

6. Some people have said that it can be easier to listen to people with Möbius if they do not see them, or if they cover their mouths. This may just reduce the distraction of looking at the face for lip movement that is not there. But there may be a contribution too from the McGurk effect. McGurk and McDonald showed in 1976 that when you watch a face and the person is making one sound or phoneme but you hear a different one, then you perceive a third independent one. For example a seen 'ga' and a heard 'ba' can be perceived as a 'da'. This shows that auditory perception is dependent on both sound and vision. Possibly in those with Möbius, who often find it difficult to make speech sounds, the absence of a movement produces a 'negative' McGurk effect [McGurk and MacDonald, 1976].

   (I was once taking a history from a lovely old lady when a junior doctor, and she said she was sorry but she couldn't hear me without her glasses, and gave me a pitying look in response to my scepticism. She put her glasses on, and the hearing aid concealed within them, and I took her history.)

7. A friend is an astronaut who does not suffer fools gladly. For one mission aboard the Space Shuttle she had made a series of cards for her various moods, from

happy to fed up, angry, and ready to breathe fire. They had to assemble a hugely complicated piece of kit, which no one on board thought worth the trouble. As they did so, Mission Control asked various questions about how it was going and were greeted by Marsha holding up increasingly unhappy cards ending with a skull and crossbones, after which Houston wisely kept quiet. I have long thought that such emotion cards would make a fortune as an executive Christmas present.

8. Steve Clark from the UK was body brushing's initial practitioner until his early and unfortunate death. More recently it has been picked up by Jenn Clarke as a treatment for dyslexia, dyspraxia, attention deficit and attention deficit and hyperactivity disorders, educational or behavioural difficulties, balance or coordination and Möbius syndrome, see www.bodybrushing.com. It involves sessions of gentle brushing of the skin over the body, arms, and face, which is claimed to be therapeutic both for calming down and in some cases for neurological improvement. In scientific terms its rationale and efficacy are unproven, but many people have found it useful. Like many treatments involving personal interrelatedness and possible therapeutic touch, it may be tapping into social and affective functions of the nervous system, which are poorly understood. It may also benefit from the fact that some people with Möbius have severe weakness of facial movement rather than complete paralysis which can improve as they grow.

(One person with Möbius told me that the most useful thing Steve had taught him was to eat bananas to avoid his energy plummeting during the day.)

9. Sara Rosenfeld-Johnson, of TalkTools, Tucson, Arizona (info@talktools.net).
10. For a good discussion of the body image see [Gallagher, 2005].
11. One person who went blind as a young man said that the lucky ones were those who had always been blind and so were unaware of what they had lost. [Cole, 1998].

Chapter 4

1. Valerie Gray Hardcastle [1999] relates how pain in children is often underestimated. Indeed, not too long ago, there was debate as to whether young children and babies actually felt pain at all.
2. Cartesian dualism has been attacked for many years, particularly by an increasingly vocal and supported tradition of philosophy stressing the importance of the body and of embodied and social interactions with the world. For a recent account of such work see Gallagher [2005].
3. Samuel Beckett wrote in similar terms about being unable to stop in *The Unnameable*.
4. The masseter transfer involved taking a small part of the jaw-closing muscle in the cheek (being a mastication muscle rather than one of facial expression, it is supplied by a different cranial nerve and is unaffected by the Möbius syndrome) and moving it to the edge of the mouth. The idea was that when she clenched her jaw, in addition she would lift her mouth at the corners, in a sort of smile.

5. Celia is being more truthful than she realizes. She is using the masseter transfer in an appeasement or social smile, which is very different to the unconscious enjoyment smile, which also involves movement around the eyes, and which she does not have.

6. Wittgenstein wrote, 'Don't think, look.'

7. Donna Williams, who has an autistic spectrum disorder, wrote of her own realization of what faces did when, as an adult, she saw a child.

'I watched the ease with which she hugged her parents. I watched the expression on her face… What she did was not just for image, for acceptance. It was not out of insecurity to make sure they would still like her. There was something happening for her that affected not her expression but the change in her expression. What she did had come from feelings, and the change in her expression seemed like a dialogue between her and her parents.'

[Donna Williams, 1994]

8. Duncan and Clare's narrative condensed from [Cole, 1998], with permission from The MIT Press.

9. Wittgenstein [1980] wrote much about facial expression and its social context, 'Would [a] fixed smile really be a smile? And why not? – I might not be able to react as I do to a smile. Maybe it would not make me smile myself.'

10. We became inseparable friends for the next decade.

Chapter 5

1. Lizzie's use of that term is interesting. Some people with Möbius (and other conditions) view themselves as 'disabled' and are comfortable with that terminology, while others are not, thinking it at best an inconvenience and at worst a way of marginalizing and defining difference.

2. Having movement on one side only means that when Lizzie smiles or makes any movement of the face, the asymmetry is accentuated, with the upward movement of the mouth during smiling, for instance, being seen only on one side. This means, in turn, that Lizzie tries not to move her face much at all. Though her Möbius is one-sided only, it imposes on both sides and on her, making her reluctant to let her face go and express one-sidedly, so drawing attention towards herself.

3. Henrietta commented;

'This is the all-life consequence of having a visible difference. However on top of the world you feel mastering social skills and managing other people's reactions, a comment, an attitude, a mode of behaviour, can come from nowhere and at any time of your day, week, or life and it will knock you off your perch.'

4. With any impairment it must be difficult to know which part of you is due to it and which to yourself. How to distinguish your own thoughts and feelings and

those imposed by the condition? At the beginning of *An Anthropologist on Mars,* Oliver Sacks [1995] quotes (or attributes) William Osler, 'Ask not what disease the person has, but rather what person the disease has.' In truth, however, these two are not separate but, rather, intertwine in a myriad of ways, especially when the condition is present from birth. Impairment might disguise, prevent or impair some aspects of a person's individuality. Lizzie felt that her Möbius was but a part of her yet, for some, it defined her.

5. This is, in part, because she is remembered by more people than she remembers. In some people with Möbius it can also happen because of their poor eyesight.

Chapter 6

1. This chapter is abridged and reproduced from [Cole, 1998]. I am grateful to The MIT Press for permission.

Chapter 7

1. The combination of facial paralysis, eye movement deficits, and ptosis (dropping of the upper eyelid over the eyes) has been described with a translocation of chromosome 1q22. Developmental delay is described as minor, but there can be heart problems too. That Alison's case does not fit neatly into the cases thus described most probably reflects inadequacies of classification as yet. (www.neuro.wustl.edu/neuromuscular/nanatomy/vii.htm#mobius).
2. She only had speech therapy at 16.
3. Many of these certificates were hanging on the walls of their sitting room.
4. Peggy showed me a lovely photo of Alison aged 5, sitting looking at a small flower she holds in her lap. Taken side on, she is looking down. It is the one photo when her eyelids are not obscuring her vision and she is not holding them up.

Chapter 8

1. The Gramercy Park Hotel when it was old-fashioned and cheap.
2. This was probably a tensilon test for myasthenia, a routine procedure usually.
3. Wittgenstein, quoted in [Monk, 1990].
4. Rumsey, personal communication, but this work is discussed in [Rumsey and Harcourt, 2005].
5. For many years a professor at Langley Porter Neuropsychiatric Institute, Paul Ekman's basic research has been on emotion and its expression. He has published over 100 articles and 10 books. He was named by the American Psychological Association in 2001 as one of the most influential psychologists of the 20th century, based on publications, citations, and awards.
6. Some years ago, my colleagues and I published a paper [Calder *et al.*, 2000] on the recognition of facial expressions of emotion in others in three people who live with Möbius, and found that this was normal, in contradistinction to previous work. But those with Möbius did appear to have some problems when asked to

describe what faces did to express emotion. This will be considered in more detail in the final chapter.

7. Mike Oliver made exactly the same point to me, in almost exactly the same words.

8. At one Möbius meeting I had spent my time with adults discussing their experiences. At the end of the meeting it was a great privilege to be awarded an 'Honorary Möbian' certificate.

Chapter 9

1. Outside Harry Potter.

2. I once said to a politician who was blind from birth that when he was being interviewed on television he often looked austere and cerebral. He replied that when he was thinking about politics, he was not in the face. When he was in a more social situation he did try to inhabit the face emotionally and communicate more through it.

3. 'Consciousness in another's face. Look into someone else's face, and see the consciousness in it, and a particular shade of consciousness. You see on it, in it, joy, indifference, interest, excitement, torpor and so on.' [Wittgenstein, 1981].

Chapter 10

1. Michael Frayn [2006] has written about the importance of narrative in our understanding of the world and of ourselves:

   We understood Genesis long before we understood *The Origin of Species*... We have to know what real death and grief are before we can understand *Hamlet*.

   But then he continues;

   Oh sure, and it works the other way too. We have to see *Hamlet*, or something like it, before we know quite what we're feeling about our own stepfather.

   Eleanor was similarly using emotion within music to guide her to an understanding of emotion in general. The retreat of many with Möbius into literature and music may be in part for escape, but we all use art, in part, to enable us to understand ourselves more.

2. Sander Gilman [1999] has written of how people with facial visible difference just want to pass with their peers and not draw attention to themselves.
   This may be true up to a point. Henrietta commented;

   'I wonder about this. I think you do want to merge in with others as you are coming to terms with it, learning to be accepted. But now I am perfectly happy to stand out and to be the centre of attention. I am not very good at being quiet in a group any more.'

   Perhaps this reflects some of the problems of putting people together and presuming a single view. Some people with a disability insist on being called a person with, say, spinal cord injury, to avoid them being identified by their problem.

Others are happy to be called tetraplegic, linking identity with the condition. We use 'person with Möbius' and 'Möbian' in that spirit.

3. Samuel Beckett's disembodied narrator of *The Unnameable*, living without movement or action has no choice but to go on too.

4. Choice, freedom to choose one's actions, friends, clothes, job, etc., are all reduced by impairment. Merleau-Ponty [1962] meditates on the importance of choice:

Freedom is doing… freedom is to have room in which to move… real choice is that of whole character and our manner of being in the world.

Those with Möbius must accept the friends who will befriend them, the shoes that will fit, and games people pick them for. Their ability to impose themselves on the world may be reduced by their problems but also by others' perceptions.

Chapter 11

1. Because the face does not wrinkle, it can be quite difficult to know the age of a person with Möbius.

2. In fact, several people said that after talking, and seeing their finished piece in the book, they had gained something from the process themselves, an understanding which was in some way therapeutic. The first lady I saw without facial expression, due to a rare stroke rather than Möbius, actually asked me to write; 'Tell, please, tell,' since her experience was so isolating and misunderstood by those around her.

3. Some years ago, I was making a film about a friend, Ian, who had lost cutaneous sensation and movement/position sense. One day we got up at 4 a.m. in Chicago to fly to New York to interview the person who had first described the syndrome, after a quick lunch. He met us at the lobby of the hospital in the Bronx and asked casually if we would be prepared to chat to a few doctors beforehand. Of course, we agreed, and were shown into a packed lecture theatre with round 100 doctors and neuroscientists who had been waiting for us to arrive.

I had never placed Ian before a medical audience, knowing his reticence, so I spent the time trying to protect him without seeming to take over. In the corner of my eye I could see the cameraman discussing with the director whether we should film it, since they could see our discomfort. After the lecture, and after lunch, we got a great interview.

4. The daughter of a friend joined a new school and pulled the same stunt in her first week. Unfortunately, the head was not amused when he saw (all of) her, aged 16. He was even less amused when it was picked up by the national press with a typical underplayed headline along the lines of, 'Millionaire's daughter in posh school nude dash shock.'

5. Möbius can be associated with various muscle problems.

6. Haruki Murakami [1987] wrote:

'I had been playing from the time I was 4 years old, but it occurred to me that I had never once played for myself. I had always been trying to pass a test or practise

an assignment or impress somebody... after a certain age you have to start performing for yourself. That's what music *is*.'

7. Christopher Reeve wrote of the 'numb zone' when, as a tetraplegic unable to move
   or feel below the neck, he was not being stimulated and how, then, his mind
   would drift off into an almost unimaginable boredom. One imagines that
   experience may also occur in others with neurological impairment.

Chapter 13

1. Not being able to walk is the most obvious aspect of spinal cord injury looking
   from the outside. But, from the inside, bladder and bowel control, and pain,
   are equal or greater medical problems, together with lack of independence and
   work.
2. Here it is as though the narrator thinks pain is easily seen on the face.
3. 'Without movement of the eyes in the head I cannot fix on things going past the
   train as it speeds up. Instead of the rapid eye movements others have then I just
   see a blur and so try not to look outside.'
4. In one sample, 74% of the sample reported sleep problems, daytime sleepiness,
   and a condition called cataplexy. Sleep quality was poor, with frequent arousals
   and sleeping too lightly. Excessive daytime sleepiness caused persons to fall asleep
   with monotonous everyday circumstances. An increased incidence of other sleep-
   related problems, called parasomnias, including sleep talking, sleep jerking,
   restlessness, sleepwalking, sleep sweating, snoring, and breath holding, have been
   described in Möbius syndrome. These often occur during rapid eye movement
   (REM) sleep and are then termed an REM sleep behaviour disorder (RBD). Cases
   of cataplexy have also been described, in which subjects suddenly lose all muscle
   tone and so fall down, often at a time of strong emotion, sometimes injuring
   themselves as they fall [Anderson *et al.*, 2007; Parkes, 1999; Tyagi and Harrington,
   2003].
5. We are not aware of figures on suicide amongst those with Möbius. Anecdotally,
   people with Möbius have told me of cases, often in the early adult years, when
   people are often most vulnerable.
6. Rather than dismissing the placebo effect, Nick Humphreys [2002] has discussed
   how it might be useful. In a social world and before effective medicine, he
   suggests, to mount an immune or other response to a malady required some cost
   to the person. It makes some sense to gain the support and encouragement of
   authoritative figures to help oneself in such circumstances.
7. 'The way you look' is, of course, ambivalent. For those with disfigurement there
   are problems in being looked at and in looking at others.
8. What to call people with unusual appearance is a constant problem. Changing
   Faces settled on disfigurement as a term that is widely used and accepted, though
   they would prefer a more neutral expression like visible difference. We have
   followed their lead.

9. A health-care worker, who had been seeing patients with Möbius and other cranial developmental problems for over 30 years, once said to me that of all of them Möbius was the most difficult for her to get inside.

10. This is not as fantastic an idea as at first sight. Evolutionary psychologists have suggested that first-look attraction suggests a relationship between face and reproductive success.

11. In her account of resilience in Möbius, Meyerson [2001] writes of the 'hide and seek' mode in relationships that people with facial difference sometimes develop. They may isolate themselves from rejection and yet yearn to be accepted.

12. Support from parents, relatives, and friends is obviously of huge importance. But, equally, some young adults may use parents as a shield and asylum. The need is to retain that support while moving people outwards to a more social existence. The balance for parents between offering support but also encouraging independence must be very difficult.

13. One parent once told me that watching someone with Möbius was like a movie compared with a photograph of everyone else. What she meant was that one could take in much about a person from a snap shot, but that to get the same from a person with Möbius you needed a much longer time. Similarly, people with Möbius might benefit from being given a little more time to express themselves.

Chapter 14

1. The term 'learning difficulties' is synonymous with 'mental retardation', which is used in some countries. To prefer the former is not simply political correctness. By focusing on the problem they have, rather than presume an underlying cognitive problem, seems more correct as well.

2. Wittgenstein [1981] observed,

Consciousness in another's face. Look into someone else's face, and see the consciousness in it, and a particular shade of consciousness. You see on it, in it, joy, indifference, interest, excitement, torpor and so on. The light in other peoples' faces. The absence of this light does not necessarily reflect internal absences. For instance, some people with Parkinson's Disease can lose facial animation and be thought depressed and dull.

3. Personal communication.

4. Some of these patients were associated with the drug misoprostol, and may form a different population.

5. Lecture at Moebius Scientific Meeting, Bethesda, Spring, 2007.

6. See [Miller et al., 2005]. In this sample are subjects with Möbius from Sweden and from Brazil. In the Swedish study, 7 out of 22 subjects fulfilled criteria for autism; they were all also mentally retarded (sic). The Brazilian sample was from 28 subjects, of whom 17 had been exposed to misoprostol and 26 were evaluated for autism. Seven met the criteria for autism or an autistic-like condition, of whom four had been exposed to the drug. In this sample 14 were mentally retarded.

7. [Trevarthen, 1979] One cannot but be aware that mirror neurone function may be involved, but also that might be different systems for emotional action, i.e., gesture and facial expression, compared with that for instrumental action and locomotion.

8. For a discussion of looping between people see [Hacking, 1995].

9. Lecture at Moebius Scientific Meeting, Bethesda, Spring, 2007.

10. [Piaget, 1959, p. 40]. The use of the term 'autistic' for this early period of development in children, a pre-theory of mind stage, predates the use of the term for those individuals with a problem in this area; when Kanner (and Asperger) described pathological, asocial children and termed them autistic, so the word itself became 'pathologized'.

11. [Vygotsky, 1986]. Vygotsky, (1896–1934), was a Russian neuropsychologist (and polymath) and not without courage. At a time when Russian, and Western, brain science was dominated by behaviourism, he told the Second Psychoneurological Congress in Leningrad, in the 1920s, that scientific psychology cannot ignore the facts of consciousness. This was revolutionary at the time. Even until recently, in the West, consciousness was not a word that could be used in neuroscience. In talking of consciousness he was not being remotely reductionist; he was interested in the origins of higher forms of human consciousness and emotional life rather than behavioural acts so that for him culture and consciousness was a legitimate subject for inquiry.

    He also suggested that the origin of consciousness itself was through relationship with others, i.e., it was social. 'The mechanism of social behaviour and the mechanism of consciousness are the same... We are aware of ourselves, for we are aware of others, and in the same way as we know others; and this is as it is because in relation to ourselves we are in the same [position] as others are to us.' [Quoted in Alex Kozulin's introduction to Vygotsky, 1986].

12. David McNeill [2005] discusses Whorfian ideas in relation to children's development in Chapter 6 of his book, *Gesture and Thought*.

13. [Vygotsky, 1986, p. 249]. He also suggests that the relation between thought and word is not fixed,

    The relation of thought to a word is not a thing but a process, a continual move-ment back and forth from thought to word and from word to thought. In that process, the relation of thought to word undergoes changes that themselves may be regarded as development in the functional sense. Thought is not merely expressed in words, it comes into existence through them.

    More recently, similar ideas have been expressed by Dennett [1991].

    Language infects and inflects our thought at every level... The structures of grammar enforce discipline on our habits of thought... the sneaking suspicion that language isn't something we invented but something we became.

    This quote taken from a wider discussion of these concerns in [Frayn, 2006].

14. 'The flow of life that social interaction involves' echoes Wittgenstein. Much of his early work as a philosopher was concerned with what language could and could not communicate. Yet he was forced to alter this way of thinking by a Neapolitan, Piero Sraffa, who was an economist at Cambridge. As Monk relates in his biography of Wittgenstein.

    'In the preface to the [*Philosophical*] *Investigations* [Wittgenstein] wrote, 'I am indebted to this stimulus for the most consequential ideas of this book.''

    Wittgenstein was insisting that a proposition and that which it describes must have the same logical form (or grammar). Sraffa made a Neapolitan gesture – brushing his chin with his fingertips and asked. 'What is the logical form of that?' This led Wittgenstein to abandon his earlier idea that a proposition must in some way be a 'picture' of the reality it describes. Sraffa gave him an 'anthropological' way of looking at philosophical problems, looking at language in the social stream of life in which it was used, rather than in a more theoretical cognitive way.

    Equally, by using a gesture, albeit one made without accompanying language, Sraffa showed that communication is not solely through speech but that language needs embodiment through gesture as well. [Monk, 1990].

15. The title *Gesture and Thought* of McNeill's book, of course, echoes that of Vygotsky.

16. There is evidence that children with spinal muscular atrophy type II, who cannot walk or stand, and so live from wheelchairs, are precocious at grammar. Sieratski and Woll [2002] suggest that, 'In place of a world they cannot reach they are building grammar, while able-bodied children engage with the physical environment.'

    This raises the possibility that some children with Möbius may be precocious readers, 'conversing' with characters in their books in a manner with which they are unable to converse in their daily lives because of their somatic problems.

17. Eric Kandel [2006] has written on this recently in *In Search of Memory*.

18. There is another anecdotal observation, which may give credence to the idea of motor programmes underpinning perception.

    Some years ago, I worked with David McNeill and Shaun Gallagher with a subject, Ian Waterman, who has lost all sensation of touch and movement/position sense from below the neck. Ian was initially unable to control movement at all. Slowly though, by thinking about movement and looking at the moving body part he relearnt to feed himself, work, and walk. But then he realized he did not gesture and so, when talking, felt passive and different. So he taught himself to gesture, thinking about it as he talked, so fooling other people into believing that his gestures were normal. More recently many of these gestures now seem to be automatic.

    Since he cannot feel his gestures, any feedback he has must be through looping through others or from visual feedback. But during one experiment we allowed Ian to move his arms without him seeing. When talking with others he began gesturing before he was aware of so doing. This elaboration and planning of gestures within the brain, of which he was not aware, may have been facilitating expression and speech.

19. Manfred Holodynski, a developmental psychologist, following Vygotsky, goes further [Holodynski and Friedlmeier, 2005; Mechsner, 2006]. He suggests that emotions evolved primarily for communication rather than experience, and are a kind of protolanguage acquired in similar ways to language and are learned by shaping and refining so-called proto-emotions.

'If we consider adults alone, we might come to believe that the essence of emotions is that they are inner, private feelings. However, if we have a closer look at children, a quite different picture seems to emerge.'

The baby cries – and father brings the milk bottle. The baby smiles – and mother smiles back, knowing that the child is well. By expressing his or her emotions, the baby manipulates, commands, and controls her caregivers. Inner feelings would have no effect and so communication seems the only biologically plausible function of baby emotions.

Holodynski suggests that a baby has to learn to use his or her emotions in this way. The newborn, not knowing this, has only 'proto-emotions' that are only vaguely related to the occasion and context. Only a few global emotional qualities are roughly recognizable in the face, voice, and body movements; endogenous well-being, discontent, interest, startle.

These proto-emotions develop into emotions through communicative exchange with caregivers. Parents recognize the needs of their baby, but also play emotion exchange games with them. 'The baby may display a diffuse expression of well-being, which is answered by the mother with a clear smile, which might then in turn be imitated better than before by the child, and so on.' Such facial dialogues teach the child to develop, step by step, clearer emotions, and to recognize and signal better, and more distinctly, their causes and aims. This is why he suggests that neglected children develop neither clear emotions nor secure interpersonal relatedness.

Expression changes with age. Toddlers display emotion strongly in social context and when alone. Between 7 and 9 years of age, the children develop the miniaturization of emotion expression more typical of adults. Holodynski investigated the reaction of children of different ages to finding an empty box that they had expected to contain a sweet: 'Toddlers seemed always quite disappointed, whereas schoolchildren showed their disappointment only if adults were present, but not, or much less, when alone.' When asked, these older children said that they had been disappointed, nevertheless.

He interpreted this by analogy to Vygotsky's theory of language acquisition in children, going from a social situation to an internalized state allowing more complex thought. Emotions were initially, through bodily feelings, designed for communication of needs; then communication of these could be regulated socially and, in parallel, internalized to allow emotional experience and simulations to take place 'offline' from social interaction. This is another, independent, account of bootstrapping emotional experience to that advanced in this chapter.

We are very grateful to Franz Mechsner of the University of Northumbria for bringing this work to my attention and for translating it.

20. Classical music, particularly, seems to have evolved to be richly emotional yet independent of language, gesture, facial expression, or embodied expression, and so is ideal for young Möbians. It is a purely aural and almost disembodied form of emotional communication.

21. Arthrogryposis has an association with Möbius syndrome.

22. The cause of this weakness is unclear but arthrogryposis can be associated with muscle diseases of various kinds.

References

Adelman PK and Zajonc RB (1989). Facial efference and emotion. *Annual Review of Psychology*, **40**, 249–80.

American Psychiatric Press. (1994). *Diagnostic and Statistical Manual of Mental Disorders: DSM IV*, (4th edn). American Psychiatric Press, Washington.

Anderson K, Shneerson J, and Smith I (2007). Möbius syndrome in association with the REM sleep behaviour disorder. *Journal of Neurology, Neurosurgery and Psychiatry*, **78**, 659–60.

Bandim JM, Ventura LO, Miller MT, Almeida HC, and Costa AE (2003). Autism and Möbius s sequence: an exploratory study of children in northeastern Brazil. *Arquivos de Neuro-psiquiatria*, **61**, 181–5.

Baron-Cohen S (1994). *Mindblindness*. MIT Press, Cambridge MA.

Bavinck JN and Weaver DD (1986). Subclavian artery supply disruption sequence: hypothesis of a vascular etiology for Poland, Klippel–Feil, and Möbius anomalies. *American Journal of Medical Genetics*, **23**, 903–18.

Beebe B and Gerstman L (1980). The packaging of maternal stimulation in relation to infant facial–visual engagement: a case study at four months. *Merrill-Palmer Quarterly*, **26**, 321–39.

Beebe B and Lachmann FM (1988). The contribution of mother–infant mutual influence to the origins of self- and object representations. *Psychoanalytic Psychology*, **5**, 305–37.

Bosbach S, Cole J, Prinz W, and Knoblich G (2005). Inferring another's expectation from action: the role of peripheral sensation. *Nature Neuroscience*, **8**, 1295–7.

Briegel W (2006). Neuropsychiatric findings in Moebius syndrome – a review. *Clinical Genetics*, **70**, 91–7.

Briegel W (2007). Psychopathology and personality aspects of adults with Moebius syndrome. *Clinical Genetics*, **71**, 376–7.

Briegel W, Hofmann C, and Schwab KO (2007). Moebius sequence: behaviour problems of preschool children and parental stress. *Genetic Counseling*, **18**, 267–75.

Calder A, Keane J, Cole J, Campbell R, and Young A (2000). Facial identity and expression recognition in Moebius syndrome. *Cognitive Neuropsychology*, **17**, 73–87.

Clarke A and Cooper C (1998). *When Facial Paralysis Affects the Way You Look*. Changing Faces, London.

Cole J (1998). *About Face*. MIT Press, Boston.

Cronemberger MF, Castro-Moreira JB, Brunoni D, *et al.* (2001). Ocular and clinical manifestations of Moebius syndrome. *Journal of Pediatric Ophthalmology and Strabismus*, **38**, 156–62.

Damasio A (1995). *Descartes' Error: Emotion, Reason and the Human Brain*, p. xv. Putnam, New York.

Damasio A (2000). *The Feeling of What Happens*. Heinemann, London.

Dawkins R (2006). *The God Delusion*. Bantam Press, London.

Dennett DC (1991). *Consciousness Explained*, p. 300. Little, Brown and Co, Boston.

Donahue SP, Wenger SL, Steele MW, and Gorin MB (1993). Broad-spectrum Möbius syndrome associated with a 1;11 chromosome translocation. *Ophthalmic Paediatrics and Genetics*, **14**, 17–21.

Ekman P (1983). Autonomic nervous system activity distinguishes among emotions. *Science*, **221**, 1208–10.

Frayn M (2006). *The Human Touch*, p. 251. Faber and Faber, London.

Fridlund AJ (1991). Evolution and facial action in reflex, social motive and paralanguage. *Biological Psychology*, **32**, 3–100.

Gallagher S (2005). *How the Body Shapes the Mind*. Oxford University Press.

Gillberg C and Steffenburg S (1989). Autistic behaviour in Moebius syndrome. *Acta Paediatrica Scandinavica*, **78**, 314–16.

Gilman S (1999). *Making the Body Beautiful*. Princeton University Press.

Goldblatt D and Williams D (1986). 'I an sniling!': Möbius' syndrome inside and out. *Journal of Child Neurology*, **1**, 71–8.

Gonzalez CH, Vargas FR, Perez AB, *et al.* (1993). Limb deficiency with or without Möbius sequence in seven Brazilian children associated with misoprostol use in the first trimester of pregnancy. *American Journal of Medical Genetics.*, **47**, 59–64.

Hacking I (1995). *Rewriting the Soul: Multiple Personality and the Sciences of Memory*. Princeton University Press.

Hardcastle VG (1999). *The Myth of Pain*. MIT Press, Cambridge, MA.

Holodynski M and Friedlmeier W (2005). *Development of Emotions and Emotion Regulation*, International Series in Outreach Scholarship. Springer-Verlag, New York.

Hoyne WF, Jones KL, Dixon SD, *et al.* (1990). Prenatal cocaine exposure and fetal vascular disruption. *Pediatrics*, **85**, 743–7.

Hughes HE and Goldstein DA (1988). Birth defects following maternal exposure of ergotamine, beta blockers and caffeine. *Journal of Medical Genetics*, **25**, 396–9.

Humphreys N (2002). *The Mind Made Flesh: Essays from the Frontiers of Psychology and Evolution*. Oxford University Press.

James W (1890). *The Principles of Psychology*. Dover, New York.

Jen JC, Chan WM, Bosley TM, *et al.* (2004) Mutations in a human ROBO gene disrupt hindbrain axon pathway crossing and morphogenesis. *Science*, **304**, 1509–13.

Johansson M, Wentz E, Fernell E, *et al.* (2001). Autistic spectrum disorders in Moebius syndrome: a comprehensive study of 25 individuals. *Developmental Medicine and Child Neurology*, **43**, 338–45.

Kandel E (2006). *In Search of Memory*, pp. 340ff. Norton, New York.

Kremer H, Kuyt LP, van den Helm B, *et al.* (1996). Localisation of a gene for Möbius syndrome to chromosome 3q by linkage analysis in a Dutch family. *Human Molecular Genetics*, **5**, 1367–71.

Kubler-Ross E (1970). *On Death and Dying*. Tavistock, London.

Lundy J (1999). Theory of mind development in deaf children. *Perspectives in Education and Deafness*, **18**, 1. http://clerccenter.gallaudet.edu/products/perspectives/sep-oct99/lundy.html

Manktelow RT, Tomat LR, Zuker, RM, and Chang M (2006). Smile reconstruction in adults with free muscle transfer innervated by the master motor nerve: effectiveness and cerebral adaptation. *Plastic and Reconstructive Surgery*, **118**, 885–99.

Marques-Dias MJ, Gonzalez CH, and Rosemberg S (2003). Möbius sequence in children exposed in utero to misoprostol: neuropathological study of three cases. *Birth Defects Research. Part A, Clinical and Molecular Teratology*, **67**, 1002–7.

Mayhew ER (2004). *The Reconstruction of Warriors: Archibald McIndoe, the Royal Air Force and the Guinea Pig Club*. Greenhill Books, London.

McGurk H and MacDonald J (1976) Hearing lips and seeing voices. *Nature*, **264**, 746–8.

David McNeill (2005). *Gesture and Thought*. University of Chicago Press.

Mechsner F (2006). Die Sprache der Gefühle. *GEO* **08**, 100–28.

Meltzoff A and Moore MK (1977). Imitation of facial and manual gestures by human neonates. *Science*, **198**, 75–8.

Merleau-Ponty M (1962). *The Phenomenology of Perception*. Routledge, London.

Merleau-Ponty M (1964*a*). Eye and mind. In *The Primacy of Perception*. Northwestern University Press, Illinois.

Merleau-Ponty, M (1964*b*). *The Primacy of Perception*. (trans. C Smith), Routledge, London.

Meyerson MD (2001). Resilience and success in adults with Moebius syndrome. *The Cleft Palate–Craniofacial Journal*, **38**, 3, 231–5.

Miller MT, Stromland K, Ventura L, Johansson M, Bandim JM, and Gillberg C (2005). Autism associated with conditions characterized by developmental errors in early embryogenesis; a mini review. *International Journal of Developmental Neuroscience*, **23**, 201–19.

Möbius PJ (1888). Ueber angeborene doppelseitige Abducens-Facialis-Lähmung. *Münchener Medizinische Wochenschrift*, **35**, 91–4.

Monk R (1990). *Ludwig Wittgenstein; The Duty of Genius*. Jonathan Cape, London.

Murakami H (1987). *Noruwei no Mori*. Kodansha, Tokyo. English translation (2000) *Norwegian Wood*. Harvill Press, London.

Oliver M (1990). *The Politics of Disablement*. Macmillan, London.

Parkes JD (1999). Genetic factors in human sleep disorders with special reference to Norrie disease, Prader–Willi syndrome and Moebius syndrome. *Journal of Sleep Research*, **8** (suppl. 1), 14–22.

Pastuszak AL, Schüler L, Speck-Martins CE, *et al.* (1998). Use of misoprostol during pregnancy and Möbius' syndrome in infants. *New England Journal of Medicine*, **338**, 1881–5.

Piaget J (1959). *The Language and Thought of the Child*. Routledge, London.

Piaget J (1962). *Play, Dreams and Imitation in Childhood*. Norton, New York.

Pinker S (1994). *The Language Instinct*. William Morrow, New York.

Pinker S (2002). *The Blank Slate*. Viking, New York.

Royal College of Physicians of London and The Prince of Wales' Advisory Group on Disability (1992). *A Charter for Disabled People Using Hospitals*. The Royal College of Physicians, London.

Ruesch J (1948). The infantile personality. *Psychosomatic Medicine*, **10**, 134–44.

Rumsey N and Harcourt D (2005). *The Psychology of Appearance*. Open University Press, Milton Keynes.

Sacks O (1995). *An Anthropologist on Mars*. Knopf, New York.

Sarnat HB (2004). Watershed infarcts in the fetal and neonatal brainstem:an aetiology of central hypoventilation, dysphagia, Möbius syndrome and micrognathia. *European Journal of Paediatric Neurology*, **8**, 71–87.

Sieratski JS and Woll B (2002). Toddling into language: precocious language development in motor impaired children with spinal muscular atrophy. *Lingua*, **112**, 423–33.

Sifneos PE (1972). *Short-Term Psychotherapy and Emotional Crisis*. Harvard University Press, Cambridge MA.

Stern D (1977). The first relationship. Cambridge, MA: Harvard University Press.

Strömland K, Sjögreen L, Miller M, *et al.* (2002). Mobius sequence – a Swedish multidiscipline study. *European Journal of Paediatric Neurology*, **6**, 35–45.

Tischfield MA, Bosley TM, Salih MA, *et al.* (2005). Homozygous HOXA1 mutations disrupt human brainstem, inner ear, cardiovascular and cognitive development. *Nature Genetics*, **10**, 1035–7.

Towfighi J, Marks K, Palmer E, and Vannucci R. (1979). Möbius syndrome: neuropathologic observations. *Acta Neuropathologica*, **48**, 11–17.

Trevarthen C (1979). Communication and cooperation in early infancy. In M Bullowa, ed. *Before Speech: The Beginning of Interpersonal Communication*. Cambridge University Press.

Tyagi A and Harrington H (2003). Cataplexy in association with Moebius syndrome. *Neurology*, **250**, 110–11.

Vargas FR, Schuler-Faccini L, Brunoni D, Kim C, *et al.* (2000). Prenatal exposure to misoprostol and vascular disruption defects: a case-control study. *American Journal Medical Genetics*, **95**, 302–6.

Verzijl HTFM (2005). Möbius syndrome: a clinical, radiological, neurophysiological, genetic and neuropathological study. Doctoral thesis. Radboud University, Nijmegen.

Verzijl HTFM, van den Helm B, Veldman B, *et al.* (1999). A second gene for autosomal dominant Möbius syndrome is localized to chromosome 10q in a Dutch family. *American Journal of Human Genetics*, **65**, 752–6.

Verzijl HTFM, van der Zwaag B, Cruysberg JRM, and Padberg GW (2003). Möbius syndrome redefined; a syndrome of rhomboencephalic maldevelopment. *Neurology*, **61**, 327–33.

Verzijl HTFM, van Es N, Berger HJC, Padberg G, and van Spaendonck KPM (2005*a*). Cognitive evaluation in adult patients with Möbius syndrome. *Journal of Neurology*, **252**, 202–7.

Verzijl HTFM, van der Zwaag B, Lammens M, ten Donkelaar HJ, and Padberg GW (2005*b*). The neuropathology of hereditary congenital facial palsy vs Möbius syndrome. *Neurology*, **64**, 649–53.

Verzijl HTFM, Valk J, de Vries R, and Padberg GW (2005*c*). Radiologic evidence for absence of the facial nerve in sporadic Möbius syndrome. *Neurology*, **64**, 849–55.

Verzijl HTFM, Padberg GW, and Zwarts MJ (2005*d*). The spectrum of Möbius syndrome: an electrophysiological study. *Brain*, **128**, 1728–36.

von Graefe A (1880). In A von Graefe and T Saemisch, eds. *Handbuch der Gesammten Augenheilkunde*. Engelmann, Leipzig.

Vygotsky L (1986). *Thought and Language*, pp. 34–5. MIT Press, Cambridge, MA.

Williams D (1994). *Somebody Somewhere*. Random, New York.

Winnicott DW (1974). *Playing and Reality*. Penguin, Hammondsworth.

Wittgenstein L (1980). *Remarks on the Philosophy of Psychology*. University of Chicago Press.

Wittgenstein L (1981). *Zettel*. GEM Anscombe and GH von Wright, eds. Blackwell, Oxford

Ziter FA, Wiser WC, and Robinson A (1991). Three generation pedigree of a Möbius syndrome. *Journal of Medical Genetics*, **28**, 413–14.

Index

Note: 'n.' after a page reference indicates the number of a note on that page.